T0349370

SAS AND SPECIAL FORCES

SELF-DEFENCE

SAS AND SPECIAL FORCES

SELF-DEFENCE

A COMPLETE GUIDE TO UNARMED COMBAT TECHNIQUES

JOHN 'LOFTY' WISEMAN

amber
BOOKS

This Amber edition first published in 2024

First published in 1997 as *The SAS Self-Defence Manual*

Copyright © Amber Books Ltd 2024

Published by
Amber Books Ltd
United House
North Road
London N7 9DP
United Kingdom
www.amberbooks.co.uk
Facebook: amberbooks
YouTube: amberbooksltd
Instagram: amberbooksltd
X(Twitter): @amberbooks

ISBN 978-1-83886-455-2

Printed in China

Picture credits
Illustrations by Chris West

Photographic credits
Format (Ulrike Preuss): 10, 14, 71, 87
Format (Brenda Prince): 42
Format (Carole Wright): 54
Malvin van Gelderen: 17, 34, 47, 50, 50, 57
Image Bank: 58, 93
Joel Photographic Library (Patrick Skinner): 63, 66
Military Picture Library: 22-23
Photo Press: 31, 36, 41, 69, 81

Contents

Section One: **MENTAL ATTITUDE**

Section Two: **SELF-DEFENCE TECHNIQUES**

MENTAL
ATTITUDE

Training the mind to assess dangerous situations accurately, to

avoid confrontations and to stay alert and positive is integral to

successful self-defence. This positive mental outlook, combined

with a knowledge of self-defence techniques, will reduce the risk of

being attacked and becoming a victim.

CHAPTER 1

WHAT IS SELF-DEFENCE?

Self-defence does not just involve learning techniques – far from it. It begins with a positive mental outlook and a few simple precautions, which will allow you to anticipate and avoid potential trouble. This knowledge will also enable you to deal with trouble when it occurs.

The purpose of this book is to offer the ordinary, law-abiding citizen a series of tested and tried techniques, which will help him or her avoid becoming a victim on the streets of today's urban jungles.

Around 90 per cent of successful self-defence is to do with avoiding violence. The remaining 10 per cent depends on using physical action to combat the attacker. We shall be dealing with some defensive fighting techniques in Section Two. Getting into a fight is easy. Avoiding a fight is the difficult part. Having said that, your own mental attitude is of paramount importance both in avoiding violence and in fighting a determined aggressor.

Essentially, self-defence is keeping out of trouble, but to do that successfully you have to be aware of all the situations and circumstances in which trouble is likely to arise.

The threat We live in a world where violence and lawlessness are on the increase. Our cities are overcrowded. Many people, particularly the young, are out of work or in dead-end jobs, and most can see little light at the end of the tunnel. They are alienated from the traditional stabilising forces of family disciplines, and they are fed a TV and film diet of violence and unattainable sex, where the role models are often muscle-bound supermen, and the major motivations are greed, lust, rage and revenge. Throughout history there has always been violence on the streets, the threat of robbery and sexual assault, as well as drunken brawling.

Violent confrontations and unprovoked attacks are not restricted to the streets. There has been a general increase in attacks on people whose jobs bring them into daily contact with the public in all sorts of environments. The police are an obvious example, although they are more prepared than most of us for violent confrontation, and have been trained how to deal with it. Other people whose jobs put them at risk include social workers, doctors and nurses, shop staff, bus drivers and conductors, taxi drivers and even firemen.

The response Despite the above, the chances of being attacked are still relatively small, and can be reduced even further by a few simple measures. For example, anyone interested in learning self-defence should be prepared to spend time improving their general fitness, ideally by attending self-defence classes, or by joining a club or gym with qualified fitness instructors. If you can join a martial arts club, so much the better, but you do not have to be a black-belt master to learn the instructions in this book. As far as your mental attitude is concerned, increased fitness and physical skills will boost your self-confidence, help you to think clearly and quickly, stay aware of potential dangers, and focus your energies if the time comes for physical action. Good self-defence is about preparedness and knowledge. You have to know the mentality and probable physical limitations of your attacker. The menacing character who has obviously been sleeping rough and is now demanding money from you on the street may be a drunk or a drug addict. Check him out.

The more you study and practise self-defence, the more resources you have to bring to confrontational situations. The trained person brings fitness, strength and skill. The alert person brings knowledge of

Mental attitude

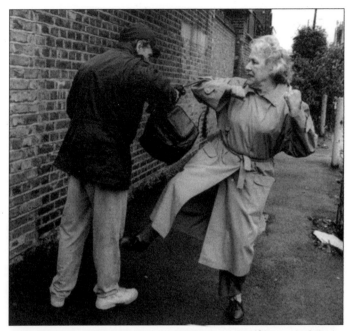

ABOVE: Mugging can be extremely traumatic for the victim. However, by following the procedures in this chapter it can be avoided with ease.

the physical environment and insights into the mentality and abilities of potential adversaries. Perhaps more important than anything else, anyone who goes into a fight knowing that he is 100 per cent in the right has an excellent chance of winning.

When to use self-defence The certainty of your moral right is a powerful weapon. Everyone has the right to defend him- or herself against physical attack. If you have done everything in your power to avoid conflict, and there is no chance of getting away by subterfuge or flight, then you have to commit yourself fully to the fight. Knowledge, skill and the conviction of your moral right will give you the determination and power to win. Some of the most ferocious fighters in both the animal and the human world are mothers with young. They do not even have to think about the rights and wrongs of their actions, they just do what has to be done.

If, however, you are not absolutely 100 per cent sure you are in the right, then you will not have that mental strength, and you may be beaten. Very many conflict situations arise out of deliberate provocation, and the fatal ingredient is often alcohol, mixed with male machismo: the need to look tough in front of your mates. For example, you are in a bar with your friends, notice that someone is staring at you, and issue the classic drunk's challenge, 'Who are you looking at?', then you have as much a chance of losing any ensuing fight as the idiot who tried to stare you down in the first place. Instead of ignoring the stare, or walking away from conflict, your pride comes into play. You do not want to look a fool or a coward in front of your friends.

To summarise, self-defence is the art of avoiding trouble. You have to know and recognise the dangers, but when, despite your best efforts, conflict is inevitable, you must know what to do. Your mind and body must be prepared to carry out the moves you have practised. Surprise and strong action combined with a strong mental attitude and a sense of your own moral right should see you through.

Self-defence for all Everyone can benefit from learning more about self-defence, and there is always something new to learn. Even professional fighters need to expand their repertoires, and think about new psychological approaches if they want to stay successful. Sometimes the strategy you employ in a fight does not work. If that happens, you have to have an alternative plan, based on your know-ledge of your own strengths and your enemy's weaknesses.

The purpose of this book is to instil self-confidence in the reader. Hopefully, one of the ways it can achieve this is by encouraging you to practise a few simple techniques which you can use when the time comes to defend yourself.

Discipline The majority of people who cause trouble are not trained and do not know how to fight. The moment you join a club and begin to learn how to fight, the first thing you are taught is discipline. You have to learn to control your movements and the emotions that can

---

Drunks and Drug Addicts

Drunks and drug addicts can be dangerous, both as perpetrators of random violence and as thieves, to gain money for their habits. Long-term drunks are easy to spot, with their puffy features, bloodshot eyes, unsteady gait and smell of alcohol. When they speak, they either slur their words or enunciate them too carefully in the attempt to sound sober. Drug addicts are harder to pin down. Amphetamine and cocaine users have enlarged pupils and uncontrolled nervous energy, and tend to gabble their words. Heroin addicts have pin-point pupils. However, in general beware of anyone who is acting in an odd manner.

Neither an alcoholic nor a junky is likely to be a match for someone who is reasonably fit and coordinated. He has probably had a bad night and has a hangover, or else is beginning to feel painful drug withdrawal symptoms. His general health is at a low level, and he almost certainly has a terrible diet. This does not mean that he is not capable of dangerous actions, but it does mean that his reactions are slow, he has little stamina, and none of the determination that you will be bringing to the situation. Indeed, your self-confidence alone will probably be enough to defuse the threat of violence.

---

govern them. You learn how to strike blows, but you also learn never to strike them in anger. You have to be disciplined in your actions, and respectful of your teachers and fellow students. The code of honour, which governs the best martial arts clubs, extends beyond the practice mats to everyday life. This is in marked contrast to the behaviour of the undisciplined street aggressors this book is designed to help you overcome. They have no training, no discipline, and are not really any good at what they do. Most of the people throwing their weight around are bullies. They can charge forward swinging when they are under the influence of alcohol or drugs, but their timing is erratic and they only have false courage.

MUGGING
Mugging is one of the oldest violent crimes known to man. It is very straightforward, being basically a matter of 'Give me your property or I'll hurt you.' The person being mugged has a fairly simple choice. Is it

worth while getting into a fight and risking injury or possible death just for the sake of a few personal possessions? The answer has to be no. Muggers often have weapons, such as knives or even guns. They also often like to work in teams. The risks attached to resisting muggers are high. Mugging is a cowardly crime, but it is also a desperate one. Don't get injured for the sake of some small change or a bit of jewellery.

Preventative measures By far the best way of dealing with mugging is to avoid it, and your preparations should start before you leave the house. First of all, do not carry anything you really cannot afford to lose. Just have the minimum of cash, and leave the flashy jewellery at home. Divide what cash you do have between several pockets. Make sure that your cheque book is separate from your cheque card. If you have many currency notes with you, fold them up and hide them in your shoe until you need them. If you are abroad, use a money belt that can be worn underneath your clothes. Wallets and handbags are particularly vulnerable, so leave them at home if you can.

In the USA many people take a special 'mugger's tax' fund with them when they go out, a few low denomination notes easily available for handing over, in the hope that the mugger will take them and run. If you are forced to hand over your bank cards, remember that you can cancel them with a single phone call. Keep the emergency number with you so that you can do that straight away. Carry a phone card. The card cancellation offices are open 24 hours a day. The more contingency planning you do before going out on the streets, the better you will feel about losing a few pounds to the mugger.

Being streetwise It is easier to avoid being mugged if you know your territory. Muggers and other opportunistic predators often congregate in airports, railway stations, bus stations and car parks, looking for easy prey. Be alert in these environments, particularly if you are not on your home ground. If you have to carry money and valuables, or are dressed up for a night out, stick to recognised routes and have someone with you. Plan your routes in advance with a local street map.

Muggers are looking for vulnerable targets, so if you are a stranger in the city be careful not to identify yourself as a soft touch. Walk with confidence with your head up. Look as if you belong. Anyone who appears hesitant and lost, trying to consult a map while struggling

Mental attitude

with bags, festooned with photographic equipment, or wearing fancy jewellery, is going to act as a magnet for muggers. If you are walking confidently and erect, with a positive manner, they will pass you by as a source of easy revenue.

SEXUALLY MOTIVATED ATTACKS

Sexual assaults vary from a surreptitious grope in a crowd to fully-fledged rape. All such assaults are an outrage, but rape can traumatise a victim and scar her mentally for life. There is no such thing as a typical rapist, just as there is no such thing as a typical rape victim. It

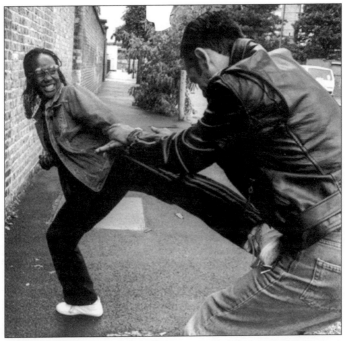

ABOVE: Avoiding sexually motivated attacks is a combination of common sense and assessment of the attacker, plus good self-defence techniques.

is increasingly realised that men as well as women are at risk, if not to the same extent. Rapists themselves are confined to no social class and no economic bracket. All they have in common is a total lack of respect for their fellow human beings.

Be prepared As with mugging and other physical assaults, prevention is better than physical conflict, but in rape there are no half measures, nothing you can give away to satisfy the attacker. A determined rapist has to be fought with total commitment. Whatever happens you are going to get abused, and you have to live with yourself afterwards, so boil up your aggression and go for broke. Many rapists are known to the potential victim, and it may be possible to deter them verbally, or bring them to their senses by shocking them, such as by throwing something through the nearest window. However, when the assailant is determined to go ahead, it is time to fight.

Fighting back Statistically, a very high proportion of women who fight back actually avoid being raped. The costs of not fighting back include humiliation, psychological damage, possibly sexually transmitted disease, including AIDS, and possible murder. A dead victim can tell no tales, and the vicious dual crime of rape and murder is all too common. Submission, in the hope of avoiding injury, gives you no guarantees at all. The best you can do is play for a little time with a diversionary tactic, to give yourself a better opportunity of fleeing, or a better opening for an effective disabling strike.

Precautions Avoiding rape situations is again a combination of common sense and an understanding of the psychology of the attacker. Common sense includes being aware of your appearance. Just as the hesitant tourist identifies himself as a potential victim to the mugger, a solitary woman dressed in revealing clothes identifies herself as a target to a rapist. Women have every right to wear whatever they want without fear of attack, but if you have dressed up for a party or a date, and have to travel alone to or from the destination, make yourself anonymous in a large coat. You can wear anything you like, including nothing, underneath.

Ideally, of course, you should avoid the need for cover-up tactics by travelling with friends or a trusted escort. It is also common sense

Mental attitude

to stick to recognised routes and avoid lonely or dark areas, such as parks and underpasses. Many women have very good street sense in this respect. If you feel uneasy about someone, that they are 'not quite right', then obey your intuition, and get away before a threatening situation can develop.

Dangers on holiday Many sexual assaults, including rape, take place when the victim is abroad on holiday. There are several factors in play here. First, you are having a well earned, relaxing time, and your guard is likely to be down. Second, if you are not aware of local cultural and religious taboos, you could be presenting yourself as someone of loose morals, and not worthy of respect. For example, northern Europeans have introduced nudism and topless sunbathing to the beaches of countries where the local residents dress from head to toe in long robes, and sex is something that does not happen unless you are married. Bare tourist flesh, and uninhibited behaviour such as wild dancing and public kissing and cuddling, can easily inflame the passions of local men. Drunkenness adds to the equation.

Some resorts have gained a reputation among tourists as partying centres, where young people feel that they are off the leash, and consume huge quantities of alcohol. On singles holidays, sexual inhibitions are often repressed by both males and females. In those circumstances, the sexual attacker may be as likely to come from your own home town as from the resort country. If you get into trouble, the local police can tend to be less than sympathetic. As far as they are concerned you will be going home in a week or two, and it will no longer be their problem. Always make sure that the people you came on holiday with know where you are, and avoid going off by yourself with strangers. Do not hitchhike, and do not accept lifts.

There is safety in numbers, as long as you know who your companions are. There have been cases where women have been assaulted or raped in crowded places, even rush-hour trains, and no-one has done anything about it. It is a terrible indictment of modern society, but selfish self-absorption, an unwillingness to get involved or disrupt one's own schedule, has made cowards of many of us. If people had a sense of moral responsibility, and were willing to team up to protect a victim against an attacker, the aggressors would have an impossible time of it. As it is, street bullies are usually confident

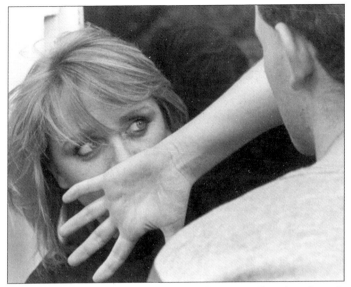

ABOVE: This book will teach you how to defend yourself against domestic violence, but your long-term defence should be to leave the abuser.

that their displays of brutality will deter all but the most determined 'have a go' heroes. We are morally obliged to answer a cry for help. By learning some of the techniques described in this book, we might be able to help save others' skins as well as our own.

Deterrents Ultimately, the woman or man faced with a sexual marauder has to depend on his or her own resources. Certainly use all means to try to deter the attack, including portable alarms, whistles and screams. Try to bluff the attacker into thinking you are compliant for a few seconds, which might give you the opening for a counterattack, but never make the mistake of thinking submissiveness will save you from injury – it won't. Fight back hard, and fight to cripple. Use anything to hand. Spray dispensers of perfume, deodorant and hair lacquer are not illegal, so use them if you can.

Theft on Trains

Subway trains are the delight of pickpockets and bag-snatchers. Rush-hour crowds are the perfect cover for a skilled thief extracting a wallet from an exposed pocket. But a few simple precautions can deter the thieves. Keep your wallet in an inside buttoned pocket if you are a man. Keep bags fastened up and in front of you, and held tight at station stops. Bag-snatchers sometimes grab and leap off as the doors are closing. Some pickpockets specialise in relieving you of your purse or wallet as you are getting onto a train. The doors close, and they are still on the platform with your property. A common scam in some countries is to have an accomplice put something nasty, such as engine grease or excrement, in a target's hair or on their clothes. In the ensuing horror and chaos, a friendly pickpocket helps to clean up the victim, or else someone else makes off with the temporarily forgotten luggage.

DOMESTIC VIOLENCE

If you are the victim of domestic violence – and this applies to men as well as to women – the appropriate level of response depends on a number of factors. In the first instance, of course, you should try to defuse the anger, or else do your best to defend yourself. Use the defensive blocks in this book, and cover up against kicks to the head or kidneys if you are on the floor. The previous history of the relationship will govern the level of any fight-back. Flight is often not an option, particularly if there are children in the house. You will already know whether this is a one-off attack, or part of a recurring pattern of abuse. If it is a frequent event, you may have a good idea of how the attack will develop – will the rage wear off quickly, or will it build up? Will it end in drunken tears and pleas for forgiveness, or will it end in rape and further punishment? You know the state of the relationship, and it may well be that you have to decide whether to try to end it. If it has happened once, it is likely to happen again. A persistently violent relationship is unlikely to get better.

Once a bout of domestic violence has ended, it is decision-making time. You will probably know whether there was a reason for the attack, or whether it was just gratuitous violence, using you as a scapegoat for something that happened somewhere else, such as being laid off, gambling losses or some other humiliation. Sexual jealousy is a frequent reason for violence, whether the jealousy is justified or not. Money troubles drive many people to despair and mindless lashing out, and alcohol is the trigger for domestic violence in a large proportion of cases.

Legal measures You have to decide whether the problem is soluble. Is a change of lifestyle feasible for either party? If it is not something you can sort out as a couple in the cold light of day, then you might have to make the break. If you consider that your violent partner is threatening you and your children with serious injury, it is possible to obtain emergency legal aid through a solicitor, and obtain an injunction banning the violent party from the family home until a court case has been heard. If this is a course you feel you may have to take in the near future, prepare yourself in advance by getting the name of a sympathetic solicitor who specialises in such cases, and talking through the logistics of such a measure.

Advice for third parties There are a number of tactical problems for third parties, such as neighbours or the police, who intervene to protect a victim in the course of a violent domestic episode. Often the first thing the police do is to grab the man, only to find themselves under attack by the woman. To defuse the situation effectively, it is necessary to split the two parties up. Do not take anyone's side. If there are two of you, one takes the woman, the other takes the man. The worst thing you can do is to grab one person in a fight, even though it may be the one handing out the punishment. If you grab the man, for example, and he starts fighting with you, and you give him a thump to cool him down, the woman could well come back into the fray, with you as her target. Don't take any chances: separate the couple. Take them to different rooms if possible, and talk them down, without allotting blame.

PERSONAL SPACE

Like most animals, humans are instinctively territorial. It is an important element of self-defence to understand this territoriality and the different forms it can take. As individuals we all have an invisible area of personal space around us. If someone encroaches on this we feel uneasy. The extent of this personal space varies according to

Mental attitude

who is doing the encroaching and the circumstances we are in. How we respect other people's personal space, and how we respond when they encroach on our space, is at the heart of successful self-defence.

Social space In our everyday activities we operate within what could be called social space. We are subconsciously aware of this social space, but if it is reduced by an encroachment, we become conscious of it. If someone comes closer than about an arm's length from us, then we feel our personal space has been invaded. This boundary varies from culture to culture. In many countries people are happy to be in crowded situations, and during normal conversations often touch one another.

Our sense of personal space is not rigid, and expands and contracts according to the social situation. We will put up with a certain amount of crowding in a queue, or in a busy street or pub, but basically we are not happy about it. As a bus fills up, all the empty double seats go first. Everyone wants to be a little island surrounded by personal space. Once crowding involves physical contact, we have a more urgent sense of invasion, because our social space has now been encroached upon. When this happens in a situation where it is totally unnecessary, the alarm bells begin to ring.

Maintaining space You can see these processes at work in a lift or on a subway train. If you are in an empty lift and someone else gets in, you move, maybe only half a pace, but enough to give you both personal space. If at the next floor several newcomers enter, there is a lot of shuffling about as you all try to redistribute yourselves around the available space. If it gets so crowded that you are almost touching one another, everyone seems to shrink in on themselves. No-one likes being crowded by strangers. If the person who enters just after you positioned himself right up against you, despite there being plenty of space, you would move away smartly, and become alarmed into the bargain. Similarly, on a subway train or a bus, if there are plenty of empty seats and someone sits right next to you, your antennae begin to twitch. You start to wonder if this person has a hidden agenda.

Respecting personal space An aggressor invades your space in order to intimidate you. Watch a drill sergeant bawling out a recruit.

Crime Statistics

There has never been a better time to learn self-defence techniques. In 1995, violent crime, meaning violence against the person, sexual offences and robbery, represented six per cent of all notifiable offences recorded by the police in England and Wales.

Robbery, defined as 'the use of or threat of force to a person immediately before or at the time of a theft', increased by 13 per cent over 1994. The police recorded a 132 per cent overall increase between 1981 and 1995.

Between 1985 and 1995, there was a 10.8 per cent average annual increase in reported rape, and a four per cent average annual increase in reported indecent assault on women.

Just over two-fifths of violent offenders in England and Wales in 1994 were under the age of 21. In 1993, one in seven men and one in 12 women between the ages of 16 and 29 was a victim of violence. (Sources: Criminal Statistics England and Wales 1995, *Government Statistical Service.* Social Trends 1996, *Central Statistical Office)*

He stands almost on the recruit's toes and shouts right into his face. The recruit has nowhere to go. The street bully tries to use the same technique. You can avoid a lot of aggravation by being careful not to invade someone's space unknowingly. Watch where you are walking. Do not close up too much on someone you are walking behind. Do not crowd people. It makes them nervous, and could trigger violence. Do not bang into people on the pavement. Avoid the bully's clumsy attempts to ensnare you into a confrontation.

Men are often at their most aware about space when they are using the stand-up stalls in a public urinal. Instinctively, you never use the stall right next to someone unless there are no others free. Similarly, you feel uncomfortable if someone uses the stall next to you unnecessarily. This is because men feel very vulnerable while urinating. If there was a sudden threat, for example, your reaction time would be slow, and you would probably end up with urine all over your trousers. Incidentally, some muggers know this, and strike when the victim is in full flow – it always pays to stay alert at all times if you have to use a public convenience.

Mental attitude

Right: SAS soldiers operate in small teams behind enemy lines. This means maintaining high levels of alertness at all times.

LEVELS OF ALERTNESS

It is possible to think about alertness as a series of levels, through which you move up and down like a driver changing gears according to traffic and road conditions.

Level One When you are at home, you are safe. You know where everything is and you are at your most relaxed. You can call this Level One. The moment you walk out of your front door you are at Level Two. You have gone up a gear, and you start to keep your eyes open. This will eventually develop into a routine. You look down to where you are treading, so as not to trip up on the pavement or tread in anything nasty. Your eyes move from the ground ahead and then back up to mid level again.

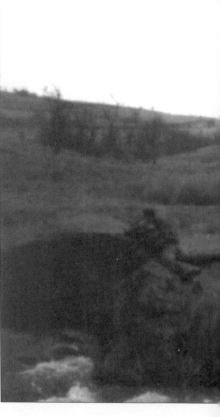

Level Two At this level of alertness, you are taking in your immediate environment with scanning glances. You look up, and to the left and right, but in a fairly relaxed way, not with a nervous intensity. Before you set off down the road, you check behind you. You keep your eyes moving, high and low, just looking around. This sort of alertness becomes second nature to people who spend a lot of time out in the wilderness, in woods and on mountains. That way they avoid tripping

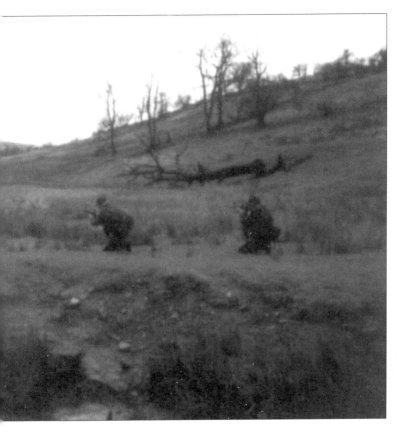

over rocks and treading on snakes, they see animal tracks and recognise birds and small creatures. It is a heightened sense of life, and it is also a way of saving your life.

In the urban environment Level Two alertness is the first stage of self-defence. Keep looking about you, and be interested in everything you see. You are finding out more about the world you live in, and you are polishing your senses. From the security point of view you do not miss anything. Look over your shoulder now and then. Look up at buildings and trees. Check the middle distance. Keep an eye on the traffic. You can make a series of mental games out of it. Analyse the world about you as you go along. Why is that man in a hurry? What happened to that car's windscreen? Is that cat going to get stuck in that tree? Is that his wife or his girlfriend? Does that house belong to a solicitor or a rock star? So many people who have a daily routine of travelling to work in the morning and then travelling home again at the end of the day complain that they are bored all the time. Yet they walk along with their heads down, thinking about their worries, fantasising about what they would like to say to their boss. Meanwhile, the world goes on all around them.

Level Three At Level Two alertness you are not going to get run over, and no-one is going to walk into you. You are also going to pick up on the situation that could bring you up to Level Three. With your eyes open, you see a gang of youths ahead of you. They are checking you out, beginning to stare. You have given yourself a little time to assess this situation by being alert, so you can cross the road. If they cross the road too, Level Three alertness will automatically kick in. Level Three focuses all your attention on the task in hand, and prepares you for flight or fight if other techniques fail. It is impossible to be at Level Three alertness from the beginning of your journey, because the secretion of adrenalin which gives you the explosive energy to flee or fight cannot be maintained for an extended period of time. The longer you maintain it, the more tired you become. Basically, you cannot walk around like a gunfighter all the time

In a slightly different scenario, if you notice that someone is following you, the thing to do is to cross the road and start walking back in the direction you came from. If the follower also crosses over, then he has shown his hand. You are up to Level Three alertness, and it is time to frustrate the aggressor by denying him the chance of attacking you while you are on your own. Head for a crowd, somewhere there is a good chance of getting help. Go into a bar. Stay with other people. Always get help whenever possible. Evasive measures which isolate you, such as running down alleyways and climbing fire escapes, are strictly for the movies. What you need most is lots of other citizens around you. However, if the situation does not allow you to seek out safety in numbers, and if you remain isolated, without an escape route, and your persistent follower has a weapon, or is threatening a sexual assault, then this is where self-defence comes in.

CONFRONTATION

The easiest way to get into a confrontation is to be drawn into a verbal slanging match. Often this can happen as a result of getting caught up in the macho staring game we mentioned earlier. Someone's eyes lock onto yours, and you stare back instead of breaking the tension by scratching your nose or looking away. If you are challenged in this sort of situation, do not give any smart answers. If someone gives you that startlingly original line, 'What are you looking at?', just say, 'Excuse me?' It does not matter if the aggressor is in the wrong, do not rise to the bait, because it will only end in violence. All you need to say is, 'Oh, sorry mate, I mistook you for someone else.' Be friendly. Sometimes it helps to smile at people. It does not matter that they may think you are a simpleton. If you say, 'Sorry,' and back off, you have demonstrated that you have no aggressive intentions. If the other guy carries on with something like, 'Right! I'm going to have you', then you know that he wants to continue the confrontation. You also know that he has underestimated you. He is at fault, and you have the element of surprise working for you. He will think you have backed down because

---

Men's Reactions to Solitary Women

Women are usually particularly sensitive to the threat of their space being invaded, because of the sexual overtones of unwelcome proximity. Men can go a long way towards reducing women's anxiety by taking care not to unwittingly become a potential threat. At night, for example, do not walk up behind women on the same side of the road if you can avoid it. On public transport, if a woman is the only passenger in your compartment or on your deck of the bus, sit away from her and where she can see you. Do not try to engage her in conversation, and do not make unnecessary eye contact. Never stare at women in any situation, and particularly avoid staring at their breasts. Never stop the car you are driving to call them over so that you can ask directions. A man in a car is particularly frightening to a woman on a lonely road.

he has succeeded in intimidating you. He does not know that you think needless violence is stupid, and he certainly does not know that you have trained and practised your moves and are confident of your physical abilities. He is going to come on to you now, but you can pick the time for sudden action, and you are going to control the fight.

Dialogue Think of the whole process of confrontation as conforming to the rule of the four Ds. The first of these is Dialogue. The whole episode begins with an aggressor challenging you verbally, and you responding in a placatory manner. You use dialogue to defuse the tension as much as possible, showing that you have no aggressive intent whatsoever. 'Sorry, mate, I thought you were someone else. Nice day, isn't it? Do you often come to this pub?', and so on.

Direction The next D is Direction. If the guy continues to come at you, say, 'Stop! Hold it!' Put your hands up at chest level with the palms open and facing outwards. You are still showing no intent whatsoever, but you are also issuing a warning. Speak in a loud voice, to draw other people's attention to what is happening. You want others to witness your actions. 'Drop the knife! Keep away from me! I don't want to speak to you. Don't come any nearer!' You have now carried out the Direction option. Witnesses will have taken note of what is happening, and this will be in your favour later on if the authorities want to know whose fault the fight was.

You have tried to defuse the situation with words, and you have progressed from there to a very firm and unmistakable verbal warning. If the aggressor makes a grab for you at this point, you are entitled to do everything in your power to neutralise his attack. You cannot afford to let him come too close before you act. Whoever gets the first punch in is ultimately going to be the winner. Once you have given him every chance to withdraw from his attack, and he still comes on, you will be foolish to wait for a single second. The strikes and combinations we demonstrate in this book, once learned and practised, are very fast and very effective. The fight should be over in a matter of seconds.

Debriefing Now it is time for the Debriefing part of the sequence. This phase involves offering support to the person who is down there on the floor wondering what hit him. Do not run away after a fight. Explain

> ## Self-Defence and the Martial Arts
> *When people have had a certain amount of training in boxing, say, or judo, in an emergency they will resort to what they have been taught. The boxer will tend to lash out with his fists. The judo expert will want to do grips and grapples. The self-defence techniques in this book are taken from many disciplines. There is some of the superb balance of tai chi, some of the more aggressive locks in ju-jitsu, some of the blocks from karate, and so on. But the self-defence taught in this book obeys no particular set of rules. Many of the strikes would get you disqualified from an organised bout. As a good rule of thumb, if something is considered to be a foul in some combat sport or other, it is probably an excellent self-defence technique.*

why you did what you did. 'I gave you plenty of warning, but you kept on coming, so I had to put you down.' By being supportive at this stage, you defuse the situation further. 'Now let's have a look at you. I'm going to stop that bleeding, it's not as bad as it looks. If that arm's fractured we'll get a medic to look at it.' Get the onlookers to lend a hand, and pass to the final D of the sequence, Documentation.

Documentation Ask around for witnesses who will be able to vouch for your version of events. 'Excuse me, sir, did you see that?' They are probably all too delighted to back you up at this point. You gave ample warning, and then when it came down to it you were swift and efficient. Then you showed a humane concern for the aggressor. Can I have your name, please?' Signed, sealed and delivered.

TO RECAP: THE FOUR Ds

• **Dialogue** Try to defuse the situation by talking reasonably and not getting into a slanging match.

• **Direction** Issue clear, firm commands. Shout 'Stop!' Most people have been exposed to some form of discipline at some time, and like a dog conditioned to its master's commands, your attacker will hesitate, even if it is only for a fraction of a second. His discipline and reactions

---

Threats

In the preliminary slanging match leading up to a fight, many people issue bloodthirsty threats that they do not really intend to carry out. 'Right, you're dead, you are. Let me at him, I'm going to kill him. I'll maim you, you bastard', and so on. Always refrain from this sort of threat. In law, if you have been heard to threaten someone with death, and then he dies accidentally in a subsequent fight, this will be used as evidence of murderous intent by a prosecuting lawyer.

---

may be fuddled with booze, or masked by drugs, but in the back of his mind the command registers, and he knows that he is in the wrong. He may well keep coming, but you have shaved a sliver off his self-confidence, and you have time to enable you to get the first strike in.

• **Debriefing** The attacker is on the floor, hurt, and you explain why you did it, and then you are supportive, treating him in a way he would never have treated you if he had won the fight.

• **Documentation** Finally, you make sure you have access to some willing witnesses in case there are repercussions.

THE SAS AND SELF-DEFENCE
The self-defence techniques in this book have been brought together from a variety of disciplines, and reinterpreted by experienced SAS personnel to suit the needs of the average citizen. In actual military close-combat situations, there is a level of violence that would be totally inappropriate in a civilian setting. Members of the SAS are taught what are called speed kills. The fastest draw, the fastest punch or strike are the ones that leave you alive and your enemy dead or maimed. In Close Quarter Battle (CQB), you use anything that comes to hand, and you move with explosive speed and aggression. The intensity of your attack or counterattack should be such a surprise that your opponent has no time to respond. In CQBs, if you do not have a real or improvised weapon, you use your body's weapons. In the military context anything goes, because your opponent is the enemy. He has to be neutralised.

This book tries to teach you some of the same techniques of speed and aggression, though not the lethal moves that are used in combat. One thing is the same, though: the faster the fight is over, the better. In the SAS, we aim for the five-second knock-down (you do not want to take any punches whatsoever).

SELF-DEFENCE AND THE LAW

In most Western countries, the law allows you to defend yourself with the minimum amount of force necessary. That is why the four Ds (see above) are so important.

Excessive force You will have warned an attacker before you put him down, and you have witnesses who will back you up. But if, after he is on the ground, you continue to kick him, punch him, bang his head on the floor, you are in the wrong in the eyes of the law. The law does not like muggers and rapists any more than you do, but it draws the line at killing them or crippling them for life. Use the minimum amount of force necessary. Of course, this will vary according to how much force the attacker offered, whether he was armed, and whether there was more than one attacker against you.

Weapons When you use some sort of weapon to defend yourself, the law is even stricter. You are not allowed to carry any sort of weapon, including things like snooker cues and baseball bats, which show an intent to use violence. You can carry an umbrella or a walking stick, because it is impossible to legislate against these. The law will come down on you heavily if you use a knife or a gun. Disabling spray canisters, such as CS gas, are also illegal in many countries. However, a woman could use a hair spray to discourage an attacker. In the section on self-defence techniques later in the book, we deal with a whole range of everyday legal items which can be used very effectively against an attacker. If, in the end, as far as the law is concerned, you have acted reasonably in defending yourself or your family, and have not pressed your advantage to the extent that you have maimed the aggressor, you should get a sympathetic hearing, particularly if you have taken down the names of a few reliable witnesses. So be aware of the laws of the country you are in, and do not forget the Documentation part of the four Ds. It could save you a lot of grief.

CHAPTER 2
POSITIVE THINKING

The correct mental attitude is absolutely essential to successful self-defence. You must learn to foster great self-belief, read a potential aggressor's body language and train your mind to overcome fear. You can even deal with pain with the right mental approach.

For successful self-defence, you need to believe in yourself. You also need to have self-esteem, which is not quite the same thing. Believing in yourself is partly about having confidence in your ability to deter or overcome an attack. You have made yourself more physically fit, and you have learned self-defence techniques and practised them repeatedly until they are automatic. You are physically prepared for self-defence, and you are confident that you can win and survive.

Self-esteem This is more to do with how you feel about yourself as a person. In a conflict, this comes into play because you know that you are in the right. This book teaches you how to act against the undisciplined, the unscrupulous, the drunk or drugged, and the dishonest, who do not play by the rules, but act according to the

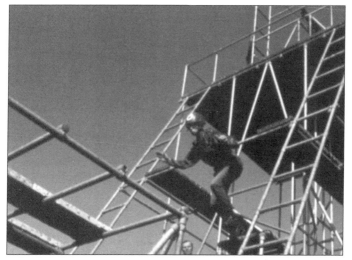

ABOVE: A potential recruit to The Parachute Regiment jumps across a gap high off the ground. Such measures are designed to test individuals' will to win.

dictates of their greed, lust, anger and stupidity. You can deal with these people if you believe in yourself and are determined to frustrate their antisocial actions. To be prepared for the unexpected attack you have to get your mind focused. It is necessary to move from a pleasant, passive outlook if you are to defend yourself from someone who is trying to violate, injure or even kill you. You must have a strong mental attitude and control your emotions. Confidence, self-belief and high self-esteem all come into this.

THE WILL TO WIN
The most basic trait in our psychological makeup is the will to live. Self-defence training is constructed from three basic elements: the will to live, knowledge and technique.

Knowledge This encompasses an understanding of the way your opponent behaves, a familiarity with the terrain you will have to fight

Psyching up in Sport

Competitive sportsmen have a great range of tricks for triggering the adrenalin that will help them to win. Some tennis players, for example, deliberately get into vicious arguments with the umpires, risking disqualification, seeing just how far they dare go. Watch professional boxers before a fight. They stand almost nose-to-nose and glare ferociously at one another, trying both to intimidate the opponent and to boost their own adrenalin. American football players huddle together before kick-off, urging each other on, slapping shoulders, whooping and yelling. Power lifters stride up and down in front of the barbell, cursing it, trying to develop a hatred of it. Before they take the stage, their coaches often slap them hard about the face.

in and the physical options it provides, also confidence in your own abilities and in your training.

Technique This is your determination, skill, energy and power in a combat situation. The foundation of the pyramid that you build with your training is the will to live.

The will to live You can have all the knowledge and skill in the world, but without the will to live you could perish. It is an instinctive quality, but we need to nourish it, consolidate it and reaffirm it for ourselves. Your opponent also has a will to live and survive. Yours has to be stronger if you are to beat him.

Once you have identified your will to live you can improve on it, changing it from a basic will not to die, to a dynamic determination to win. Your whole life comes into this. It is not merely a desire to avoid being hurt. You must bring into it your love of your family and your determination not to let them down. Bring into it all the good things that make your life worth living: friends, social life and your love of laughter, colour, music and all the beauties of the natural world.

Obviously, you do not have time to review all these things in your mind when a fight starts, but if you make a habit of analysing and articulating to yourself those things you cannot afford to lose, they will become consolidated into your will to live, and will play an automatic part in boosting your drive to win the fight. Never forget that the attacker coming at you could cancel out all those good things. If he does not kill you he might cripple or blind you, destroying your ability to support your family and enjoy your life. You must get this right in your mind. You have to know with a fierce conviction that there is no way that he is going to beat you.

Self-defence psychology The will to win is the difference between champions and also-rans in the sports world. The champion has that determination and mental ability, as well as the physical skills. All winners have it in common. Some call it having a big heart or a killer instinct. Too many people ignore this psychological element. When the fight is about to happen, you must feel 100 per cent sure that you are going to win. You build your aggression up consciously, and trigger the adrenalin rush that will see you through. It does not matter how big your assailant is, or whether he has a club or a knife. But you have to be 'up for it': in the right frame of mind. Any nagging doubts you may have, any fears about your own weaknesses, will let you down. Use your mental strength. You have practised your moves., you have assessed the weaknesses of your opponent, you have run through the likely scenarios in your mind, and you have established and pumped up your will to live. Now eliminate the doubts and fears, say, 'I'm going to win', and go for it.

BODY LANGUAGE AND SELF-DEFENCE

Academic research has shown that we communicate far more information through physical means, such as facial expressions, posture, movements and gestures, than through language. In fact, what we say may well be totally negated by our body language. The teacher may say, 'This is going to hurt me more than it will hurt you', but you are right to feel sceptical as he takes off his jacket, rolls up his right sleeve and picks up the cane with a gleam in his eye. Half the time we are not even aware of the information we are absorbing from someone else's body language, which can include things like clothing, jewellery, hairstyles and makeup, as well as their behaviour.

Signals In self-defence scenarios, both aggressor and potential victim use their knowledge of body language. In the first instance, the aggressor is seeking a target who looks like a victim. The mugger's main goal is to raise some cash, but he also has a vested interest in succeeding in his robbery and not getting hurt. If you have a timid posture and creep along the street looking fearful, he will find you an attractive proposition. If, on the other hand, you are walking confidently, with your head up, the mugger may well decide to give you a miss. Your self-defence training will stand you in good stead here, because a fit person with a good sense of his or her own body has a confident gait, relaxed and well balanced. You will also look alert, eyes checking everything out. You, for your part, have read the mugger's body language. Is he converging on you without seeming to look at you; is he concealing something in his hand; does he look confident or furtive; is he dressed for a speedy getaway; and is he cutting off any escape route you may have?

Bullies depend a lot on body language, because their aim is to intimidate. We talk of a 'swaggering' bully, and the description can be accurate. They take up too much pavement, puff up their chests,

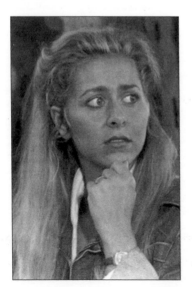

try and make their shoulders look broader. They may roll the sleeves of their T-shirts high to emphasise tightened upper arm muscles. We see the signals, as we are meant to, and give them a wide berth. We have already talked about the pub bully with a few pints in him, who uses the aggressive stare as an invitation to violence.

The eyes The appearance of our eyes and the way we use them can convey a huge amount of information. When

LEFT: If threatened, try not to look sheepish or afraid – even if you are. Try to exude an air of confidence to deter would-be attackers.

The Eyes and Character

Eye configuration can sometimes be a clue to character. When a normal person is relaxed and not looking up or down, the iris contacts the lids at top and bottom. In some people there is a space, with white showing between the bottom of the iris and the bottom lid, and this could indicate a cruel and ambitious nature. The reverse pattern, with white showing between the top lid and the top of the iris, could indicate a sadistic nature. People sometimes talk about 'mad, staring eyes', and if someone has eyes with white showing all around the iris they could be in a mentally disturbed state. Beware!

you first begin to talk to someone you make eyeball contact, and immediately there is an information exchange. If they start looking away almost at once, it could indicate that they are feeling guilty about something. If they open their eyes very wide when talking to you, they could be trying for the 'wide-eyed innocent' look. Some people blink a lot when they are nervous. Others show that they are submissive or intimidated by avoiding eye contact altogether, or dropping their head forward so that they have to look upwards at whoever they are talking to. It is also possible to harden or soften the expression by peering intently or relaxing the eye muscles.

One particular interrogation technique employed by police and military personnel uses eye movements to gauge whether the person being interrogated is telling the truth, or making something up. At first the interrogator will ask a simple question to which the subject should know the answer, but will probably have to visualise something in order to answer, for example, 'What colour is your front door?' A lot of people will look up either to the left or right as they visualise the door and the colour. So the first question has established the probable direction the subject looks when visualising a real situation. The next question will be framed to make the subject have to use their imagination, for example, 'Can you imagine your local school teacher dressed in black frilly underwear?' The eyes will almost always go in a different direction as the subject fantasises about this new image. Now, with eye-directions established for real situation visualisation and fantasy visualisation, the interrogator can ask a question for which

Mental attitude

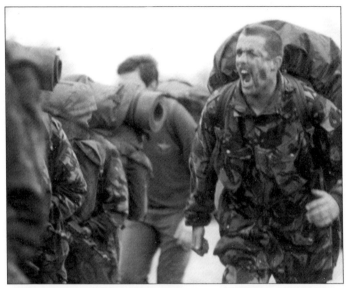

Above: A Parachute Regiment instructor deliberately being aggressive. In self-defence you must learn the difference between aggression and assertiveness.

he wants to know the answer; for instance, 'What were you doing in the street with a crowbar?' The subsequent eye movements may betray the subject as he attempts to lie, or else confirm his reply.

Facial colouring This is a good way of measuring the determination of an aggressor. The person who goes red in the face, and blusters and threatens you, saying, 'I'm going to punch you on the nose, I'm going to murder you', and so on, is not really going to do it. He would love to hit you, but he has not got the will to step over the line unless you really goad him. It should not be too difficult to talk him down. Save his face, do not touch him, back off from him, make soothing noises, 'It's all right, mate. No problems.' That way you have given him an out from his embarrassing display. He can walk away without feeling that he has lost face.

The aggressor to be really wary of is the one with the white face. His blood has drained to wherever he might need it for sudden, violent action. His pupils may reduce to pinpoints, and he will begin to look you up and down. If you are in the police or the military he is looking at the uniform, the badge of authority, not you as a person. He is deliberately disassociating you from a real person, and he is going to hurt or kill you if he can. That is when it is time to get out of the way by any means possible. The white-faced man is dangerous.

Non-violent signs When some people are nervous or upset they start to groom themselves. They straighten their tie, adjust their cufflinks, brush imaginary dust from the front of their jacket. The man who grooms himself in a confrontational situation is not going to get involved in violence. He certainly does not want to end up rolling on the floor getting covered in dust and blood. Much confrontational body language is a way of testing the water, trying to make you react so that your opponent can judge the effect they are having on you.

BEING ASSERTIVE

Rolling the sleeves up is an aggressive gesture. If you want to avoid escalating a situation, make all your movements slow when you are talking to an aggressor. Do not wave your arms about in the air. Do not crouch in a recognisably combat-ready position. However, you cannot afford to let a potential opponent take liberties. Bodily contact is strictly off limits. If he starts to jab at you with his finger, he is testing you to see just how far he can go, just how near he is to the point of no return. He may be trying to provoke you into action, but he is just as likely trying to make you back off. In this situation use Direction commands: 'Don't do that! Keep away from me! Don't touch me!' Tell him that you do not want to hit him. If he does it again, put him down fast and hard.

Language When you use Direction to control situations you are being assertive, and you have to be aware of the boundary between assertiveness and aggression, so temper your language accordingly. Remember the Dialogue rules. Always give people an out. Never threaten, and never make promises.

You never say to someone, 'Get off the grass, stupid!', even if they are in the wrong. You have called them stupid, which will inevitably

Practising Assertiveness

*Physical self-defence techniques have to be practised with a partner,
and this sort of rehearsal is equally useful with non-physical techniques.
Take it in turns to be the aggressor and the person under threat. Act
out first what it feels like to be a victim. Use a victim's submissive body
language while the aggressor uses threatening body language, invading
your space and staring you down while using verbal threats. Repeat the
exercise, switching roles. Now take it in turns to be assertive, putting
up your hands, palms outwards, and issuing loud, firm directions, such
as, 'Stop! Don't do that! Leave me alone!' Learn what it feels like to be
the one issuing the assertive commands, and the one receiving them.
The more you practice vocalising your assertiveness, the easier it will
be to carry out in a real situation.*

escalate the confrontation into a slanging match. Instead, say 'Don't
go on the grass because....' Explaining the reasons for things does
not ruffle people's pride. It gives them an out, an opportunity to behave
reasonably. When a gang of teenagers is making a lot of noise on the
street, you do not say, 'Hey, you lot, clear off!' Give them an explanation
for your wanting them to act in a certain way. Try something like, 'OK,
lads, you're making a lot of noise out there, but my mum's upstairs in
bed trying to sleep.' or 'The old man's on nights.' Most people would
understand that, and act reasonably. When you tell them to clear off
they know they are in the wrong, but will not want to be seen giving
in to an angry command. When you give them a reason, they will not
lose face by moving on.

Avoid physical contact Keep your voice down, and never lay hands
on anyone. That gives them the excuse and the motivation to grab you.
When someone is hysterical, never slap them in the face, because
they will probably slap you right back. Talk them down firmly before
trying restraint. Say 'Stop it! Be quiet!' Get through to them with your
voice. When trying to talk an aggressor out of a confrontation, do not
adopt an aggressive posture. Standing face-on with your arms folded
over your chest is aggressive, and tactically weak, as you cannot free
your arms fast to protect yourself if someone throws a punch.

If you are dissuading someone from approaching you, hold your hands at chest level with the palms outwards. This emphasises your Dialogue commands – 'Stay away!' – and your hands are where you want them if you have to fight. The open palms are a defusing gesture, showing you have no weapons. Stand obliquely to the person, and never ball your fists up, as that is very threatening. The trick is to be assertive without being threatening. People may try to distract you by waving their arms about and pointing all over the place when they talk to you. You must not fall into the trap of trying to look in every direction at once. Use your peripheral vision. Relax your eyes and look at the person in front of you at about the level of their throat.

Anger control You must always control your anger. It is anger that makes you threaten people, so that you end up painting yourself into a corner. In any situation you always want the other person to underestimate you. Lose your temper and you lose your assertiveness. You also lose your coordination, so that you start to fight with your heart instead of your brain. When you descend into a red rage all your training goes out of the window, and you revert to brute force and ignorance. Anger will destroy your fighting disciplines, and if your opponent is also trained, and has remained cooler than you, he will beat you. It is essential to give an attacker a false sense of security by controlling yourself and staying calm and collected.

OVERCOMING FEAR
Fear is a very natural accompaniment to being attacked, and everyone feels it. The man who says that he is frightened of nothing is either deluding himself or else is seriously disturbed, and should be avoided as a danger to himself and to his mates. Members of the SAS experience fear just like anyone else. In fact, anyone claiming not to experience fear would never pass the selection process.

Fear – a positive emotion It is possible to be immobilised by fear, like a rabbit confronted by a snake or a weasel, and it is this response that bullies, muggers and rapists seek in their victims. Society's attitude is that fear is somehow a negative and disadvantageous emotion, but the opposite is true. Fear is a very positive thing, and will stand us in good stead as long as we can control it and use it in our defence.

Paratroopers

The SAS are trained soldiers and paratroopers, yet even they feel fear when they, say, jump out of an aeroplane. The act itself is frightening and against natural logic. You do it because you are trained for it. You know the risks, but you overcome your fears. Apart from anything else you are in front of all your mates, and even more scared of letting them down. Overcoming the fear and jumping proves your reliability. All fears can be overcome and controlled, and this applies equally to fighting.

When you are frightened, the adrenal glands secrete adrenalin into the bloodstream. The effect of this is that, for a short time at least, you can summon reserves of energy and strength that you had no idea you possessed. It is the equivalent of a turbo charger in a car. You can run faster and lift heavier weights, and your senses are sharpened, including eyesight, hearing and sense of smell. This is a survival mechanism that all animals have, including humans, and it is the basis of the 'fight or flight' reaction to stress. The danger in a combat situation is that you may lose control of all this useful energy and descend into panic, so you have to learn how to coordinate these emergency powers. This is partly a question of focusing your mind on the task at hand. Reported incidents include grandmothers lifting cars to free their trapped grandchildren, using a desperate surge of adrenaline fuelled strength. And skinny kids have been known to throw 18-stone warders. That is the power of adrenalin. In self-defence you have to get everything in line using the adrenalin. Focusing, a sense of timing, your training – these all come together to help you make the most of your fear.

Fear control One way to have control over what is happening is to use a breathing technique. Concentrate on a point an inch or so beneath you navel as you inhale forcibly through your nose for a five count, retain the breath for a further five, and then exhale through the mouth. Repeat the cycle if you have time. This will help you to use the adrenalin reflexes. In a house fire, instead of panicking, you will have time to assess the situation and choose the right options. Your reactions are super-fast, and time seems to slow down. People who have been in a car accident where the car has rolled over have

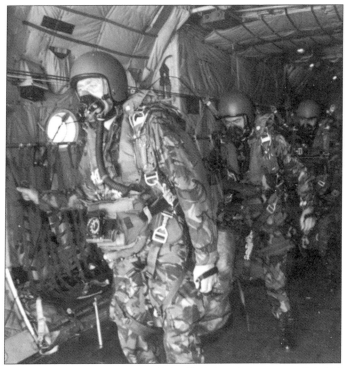

Above: Jumping out of an aircraft is illogical and dangerous. But SAS paratroopers learn to control their fear in order to carry out the mission.

described how everything seemed to be in slow motion. In this state you can see everything coming, including punches and kicks, and have time to avoid them. By controlling your breath, and focusing on what is happening as the adrenalin flows, you can work out what to do next and implement it. If you are going into a sequence of strikes which you have trained for, you focus where each strike will land. At the same time, you have to keep as relaxed as possible, to avoid your muscles tightening up and becoming too tense.

Mental attitude

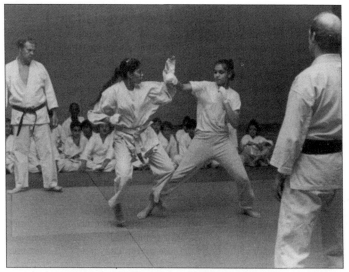

ABOVE: In self-defence, training bouts are useful for overcoming the fear of losing, as well as for sharpening up on individual moves.

The fear of losing Many people are reluctant to fight, not only because they do not want to be hurt, but also because they are frightened of losing. This sort of fear is partly due to lack of experience. The fact of the matter is that there is always someone bigger, faster and stronger than you. It is important to learn how to lose before you learn how to win. This is where training comes in. If you are used to practice bouts with training partners, you will gradually lose the fear of losing that could paralyse you in a real self-defence situation.

The aggressor on the street may well be bigger and stronger than you, but he has never practised taking a beating. He thinks he is tough, but he has no discipline. If you are a normal healthy person with training and a strong mental attitude, and you have conquered your fear of losing by experiencing what it is like to get 'stuck in', the over-confident aggressor is going to be taken aback when, instead being intimidated, you go forward and deliver an efficient strike. The bully is

---

The Adrenal Glands

The paired adrenal glands are situated like caps at the upper end of each kidney. Each consists of the adrenal medulla and the adrenal cortex. When you are under heavy stress, as with anger or fear, the adrenal medulla secretes large quantities of two hormones called epinephrine and norepinephrine to help you cope with the emergency. Your blood pressure rises, your heart rate increases, and the glucose content of your blood rises dramatically. At the same time, your spleen contracts to squeeze out a reserve supply of blood, the pupils of the eyes dilate, and the muscles that erect the hairs contract – giving rise to the saying 'My hair stood on end.' Meanwhile, the adrenal cortex secretes a different set of hormones which stimulate the conversion of proteins into carbohydrates, such as glucose, regulate the content of potassium and sodium in the body, and magnify your feelings of aggression.

---

so used to getting his own way that he will not know what to do, giving you the chance to follow through and complete your fighting sequence.

Pain and fear Finally, people are understandably frightened of the idea of pain, yet pain is a natural and useful process that prevents you from damaging your body with rash actions. It tells you something is wrong so that you can do something about it. Without pain we would accept damaging burns and wounds. If you understand pain's function in life, you can then go on to conquer your fear of it. Pain and fear go together in many ways, and both can be overcome. In a fight, when you have got your adrenalin flowing, pain is temporarily suppressed by the body. People have been shot, stabbed, even received fractures, and have not noticed until after the fight. The pain will start to come as the adrenalin returns to the adrenal glands, and then you will notice that you have the wound or the sprain or whatever. So get the adrenalin flowing when conflict is unavoidable. Control the new energy, control the fear of fighting and the fear of pain and use your self-defence techniques. At least afterwards you will be able to say, 'I did resist', and the chances are you are going to win anyway. But if you give up before you start, you are going to have to live with yourself and the knowledge that you did not try to protect yourself.

CHAPTER 3
SPOTTING TROUBLE

Prevention is better than cure, and this is as true for self-defence as it is for medicine. By using a little common sense and foresight in your everyday life and travels, you can avoid trouble and dangerous places with ease, allowing you to live a contented and stress-free life.

Provocative eyeball contact and aggressive or insulting verbal exchanges are among the main causes of fights. Both of these can be avoided as long as you remember that false pride is your biggest enemy. Slanging matches may start relatively innocuously, but they can deteriorate rapidly to the point where violence begins. In such verbal sparring it is not long before those involved are trying hard to hurt each other, probing for the raw nerve. Dragging in references to the other person's family, particularly female relatives, is a favourite ploy, as this inflames a defensive anger based on sexual pride.

AVOIDING CONFRONTATIONS
When someone locks eyes with you, the best avoidance technique is to break off the eyeball contact. Similarly, the best way to deal with

verbal abuse is not to get involved in the exchange of insults. Just say something like,'Oh, I can't discuss it now. We'll discuss it later.' It does not matter how lame you think it sounds. The important thing is to break off the contact. Let other persons say whatever they wish, and do not get rattled by their words – words will not hurt you.

Retaining control The problems sometimes arise when an insult hits a nerve, which is raw because there is an element of truth involved. If there is something in your past of which you are ashamed, and an insult dredges this up, you could lose your cool and forget that you are trying to avoid violence. You have to be impervious even to this, and use the mental strength you have gained from your training discipline to avoid a retaliatory response. Walk away from the fight. Staying out of trouble can sometimes be very hard, and you have to work at it. When the majority of people look back on a confrontation they wonder why on earth they let it happen. So never let yourself be goaded.

Distraction techniques Confrontations can often be avoided by the use of surprise tactics. Resort to any ploy that works for you, that you think is merited by the situation. If you are a convincing actor, you could try loudly crying for mercy, which might win you a few vital seconds while the aggressor or aggressors get over the shock, giving you the time to counterattack or escape. Always do the unusual and the unexpected, and play on their emotions if you can. Feigning an imminent heart attack and asking the attackers to call an ambulance, for example, is a technique that has succeeded in the past.

You could also try engaging an attacker in conversation. Talk about your health problems. Tell him you are visiting an aging relative who is close to death. It need not have a shred of truth in it. Say you are really worried by problems at work. Describe your depressions in boring detail. The point is to make the aggressor start seeing you as a human being instead of a victim, to slow up his advance on you, and make him unguarded so that you can strike or escape.

You can also break an attacker's concentration by bringing him down to earth. In one crowd fight I witnessed, a security man sobered up someone who had grabbed him by pointing out that the attacker's wife and baby were across the room. 'Hang on, your wife is over there with your baby. Go and look after your baby.' This made him think about his family, towards whom he felt protective, and broke the violent contact. Tell the other person that the police are on their way, or that his girlfriend or wife is getting very upset. The point of these tactics is to jolt the other person out of his mindless involvement in physical action, and get him to think about a different problem, something emotionally close to him if possible. These tactics can work with someone attacking you, and also if you are trying to calm down a confrontation between two or more other people.

CALMING DOWN A CONFRONTATION

If you are trying to calm down a confrontation involving other people, sit them down if you can possibly manage it. If you can stop them standing up and get them into chairs, they will not be able to fight: no-one can fight from a chair. If they try to start again, you have plenty of warning because they have to get up first. As in dealing with domestic fights, keep the protagonists apart. Turn the chairs so that they cannot see one another, and if you have a colleague to help you, put them in separate rooms while you try and talk them down and sort things out. If they are out of sight and earshot of one another, you will not have to deal with a new outbreak of verbal slanging.

Diversion tactics Be sympathetic with the person you are talking to without taking sides in the argument. Give him something to think about to help divert him. If you can make him concerned about his condition it will help. Pretend things are worse than they are. 'Bloody hell, that eye's bad! Blood everywhere! Let's get you to the hospital.' Give him a handkerchief to press over the cut. Give him something to do. Make him a bit worried and he might forget wanting to fight the other person. Creating distance between protagonists is important. As their adrenalin runs down they will start to feel exhausted. The more tired they get, the less likely it is the fight will start up again.

MAINTAINING DISTANCE

In any confrontation, you want to create distance between yourself and the aggressor so that eventually you can break off all contact by walking away, or mixing with crowds, or entering a pub or even a police station. Do not turn your back and try to run away immediately from someone confronting you, as his immediate reaction may be to

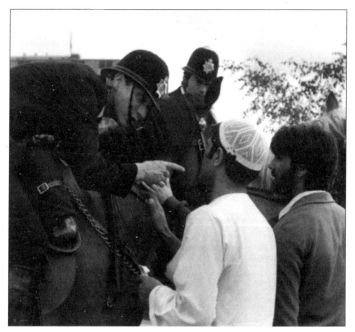

ABOVE: The police are trained to defuse potentially volatile situations. As part of your self-defence skills, you must also be able to avoid confrontations.

run after you. At all times, unless forced into close-quarter action, you should endeavour to stay at least two arms length away. If he comes forward a pace, you retreat a pace. With your hands in the ready position in front of you, palms outward, you can block punches and are ready to strike if necessary if he advances suddenly. Stay relaxed, and maintain the distance. If you tense up you will lose your timing if the fight starts. Keep trying to defuse the situation verbally, and keep moving on your feet. Move around as he does, so that you are always a safe distance away, and you can always see him.

If you sense that he is losing his aggressive momentum and the time is right to move away, do not turn your back straight away. Back

---

Escorting Strategies

If you are escorting someone who is less competent than you at looking after yourself, watch your positioning all the time in potentially dangerous areas. Watch the way VIPs' bodyguards operate when you see them on TV newscasts. Normally they walk behind, looking in all directions continually. If a door comes up they accelerate to open it, check what is beyond it, and then drop back again. Whenever unknown people approach, the bodyguard positions himself between his charge and the newcomer, changing sides frequently if necessary. Adopt the same strategies if you are looking after someone. Always look where the potential threat is coming from, and change position to block it.

---

off, staying alert and focused. Reassure him. 'All right, mate, I've had enough. I don't want to know, OK?' Continue to back away, maintaining or increasing the distance between you, and start to turn. Keep talking. Keep watching him, keep your hands up, and keep walking until you feel it is all right to make your exit without him rushing you. If he does try to grab you as you back off, still looking over your shoulder, you are in a good position to counter-strike.

BEING STREETWISE
For successful self-defence you need to be streetwise, and that means knowing your territory and knowing how to operate within it. Which areas are full of pubs and clubs? Where do most of the muggings take place? Which is the red light area? Where do the drug addicts hang out to score? Where are the big, soulless estates full of bored teenagers? Which are the streets where your car is most liable to be broken into? Where do the increasing numbers of homeless spend the night? When you are in a strange town you have to be especially wary, because you may not be familiar with these obvious danger spots. Every major city has its dodgy areas where the crime rate is high. Some of them are so bad that they are virtually no-go areas. Make it your business to know where these are, particularly if you are going to be out at night. Ask your friends who live locally. You could even ask at a police station. Then plan your routes accordingly, using a local street map. Don't leave anything to chance.

Danger areas Whether you are in a strange town or on home territory, streetwise tactics are the same. Muggings take place where the mugger can hide or look inconspicuous until he strikes, so be extra alert when you are walking in sidestreets, or in car parks, or in any dark, deserted environment. If you can, avoid them altogether. Certainly avoid public parks, wasteland, building sites, canal towpaths and river banks after dark. Be alert in the areas where the pubs and clubs proliferate, especially around closing time. Avoid areas where drug dealers operate, because addicts desperate for a fix often mug people close to the supply, so that they will not have far to go to score.

Car parks Parking restrictions in most city centres mean that the only options available if you drive into the city are parking meters with limited time availability, or multi-storey car parks. The multi-storey car park could have been custom designed for ambush and robbery. It is usually poorly lit and deserted, and its concrete pillars, stairways and ranks of cars provide the perfect cover for marauders. Muggers would far rather confront you in this sort of environment than on the streets in the centre of town where there are plenty of people around. This is their sort of territory, and they choose it for the advantages it gives them over you. The best strategy is to avoid multi-storey car parks altogether at night by taking a taxi. That way you bypass the muggers, and your own vehicle is less likely to be vandalised and robbed.

Deterrents Give yourself as many advantages as possible over potential attackers when you are out at night. Keep up with your training disciplines, and also carry a walking stick. Hand alarms and shrill whistles can be useful to halt an attacker for a second or two if they are really loud, but do not bank on anyone taking any notice in noisy areas. A dog can be a good deterrent if it is protective and brave. A bright torch can dazzle, and can also be used as a legitimate weapon as long as you have a genuine, non-violent reason for carrying it. Wear clothing which will not impede your movements and which cannot be used against you – a scarf can be used to strangle you for instance, as can a hooded jacket. If it comes to a fight, sturdy lace-up shoes are best for effective kicking. Slip-ons can fly off.

In all environments where attack is a possibility, remember that the person on the high ground has the advantage. Stand up on the

Mental attitude

kerb if a potential attacker is in the road. If there are stairs nearby, get up on those so that you are looking down at your protagonist. This gives you a psychological advantage which might deter him, and in a fight gives you a physical advantage. If an attack develops, try and put an obstacle, such as a litter bin, between you and the attacker. Use anything loose and portable, such as traffic cones and fire extinguishers, as a shield against weapons. Wherever you are, make a habit of looking around you and checking for escape routes should problems arise. This applies indoors as well as outside.

Positioning yourself strategically in a room is all part of being streetwise, so make sure you have access to the door if it is the only

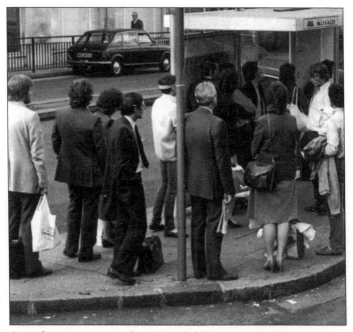

ABOVE: Our streets are usually very crowded. It pays to stay alert when you are travelling on foot, to keep a lookout for potential trouble and aggressors.

one. On the street, do not let people come up close behind you. If you are with friends, you can all keep a lookout. In an emergency, you can stand back to back if there is more than one attacker.

STREETCRAFT

Streetcraft is one of the ways you give yourself an advantage over the opportunist attacker, and the core of it is the elimination of any element of surprise he may be hoping for. When walking down lonely or dark roads, for example, be aware of road junctions up ahead of you. Someone crouching low just around a corner is invisible to you if you are on the same side as the junction, so walk on the other side well in advance. If someone is lurking around the corner, you have given yourself the advantages of time and distance. You cannot be taken by surprise, and an attacker will have to cross a stretch of open road before he can reach you. You have time to react to an attack. You have seen the man with the baseball bat, and you are switched on and focused, with all your training and preparation coming into play.

Anticipating danger The same positioning principles apply if there is a steep curve in the road ahead. Always position yourself in advance so that you will be on the outside of the curve. That way there will be no surprises. Make this second nature. Cross over if there is an area of dense undergrowth on one side which could hide an attacker. Look up as you come to footbridges, and stay clear of the stairs leading up to them. Avoid underpasses if you possibly can. Muggers at both ends of an underpass have you trapped. At night and in bad weather they are shelters for vagrants, some of whom may be alcoholics and drug addicts who may operate in gangs.

Rural areas The roads and lanes in rural areas often do not have footpaths. Never walk on the side of the road which enables cars to come up behind you without you watching them, because an attacker could suddenly pull across at an angle in front of you and trap you by throwing the doors open. You could then be dragged into the car by the driver's accomplices. So walk to face the oncoming traffic, giving yourself time to react if anything starts to happen. Walking to face the oncoming traffic is generally safer anyway where there are no footpaths, giving you time to leap out of the way of careless drivers.

Mental attitude

Anyone carrying a handbag or other shoulder bag should walk facing the traffic and also have the bag on on the side away from the road, to forestall snatch thieves on bicycles or motorbikes. On occasions, where a road is flanked by trees and shadowy hedges, it may be better from a security point of view to walk in the middle of the road, listening out carefully for traffic approaching from behind.

High-rise flats These are often stalking grounds for criminals, particularly where they are semi-derelict, in run-down areas. If you have to visit such a block for any reason at night, take a friend with you, or else be especially alert. Like multi-storey car parks, they provide would-be attackers with ample hiding places, such as stairways, corners and landings. Very often corridor and stair lights have been smashed, and muggers can also take bulbs out and immobilise lifts to give them an edge. Lifts themselves can be very dangerous. Check them before getting in, and watch out for someone leaping in at the last moment as the doors close. Do not forget it is possible for an attacker or attackers to get in with you at any of the floors.

GANGS AND DRUNKS

A lot of violence occurs at or around throwing-out time at pubs and clubs. This is when the aggravation that may have been building up at the bar suddenly bursts out as the drinkers hit the fresh air. The biggest danger for casual passers-by is probably getting caught up in someone else's fight, so steer clear if you happen to be in the immediate vicinity. Whenever possible, avoid taking public transport immediately after closing time – drunks may become aggressive when the buses and trains fill with people.

Dealing with gangs Avoid gangs of rowdy drunks if possible. They are likely to be the ones who have been left without a partner at the end of the night. They are jealous and angry and looking for fights. If you are with your girlfriend or wife, and have to walk past an aggressive-looking group, a good ploy is to brief your partner to loudly give you a hard time. 'You've been drinking again, haven't you! You said you'd be home by eleven. Have you any idea how hard it is getting the kids to bed on my own?', and so on. You will probably get a bit of sympathy: 'Leave him alone, he's got enough trouble as it is.'

Alcohol

Drunkenness is the major ingredient in a very high proportion of violent incidents. In the first place, it fuels the aggression of potential attackers; it clouds the judgement of potential victims, and makes them appear vulnerable to predators. In 1994, a quarter of all men and an eighth of all women drank above the maximum sensible level of 21 units of alcohol. Among 18 to 24 year olds, a third of men and a fifth of women drank over the sensible level. Six per cent of men and two per cent of women drank at a level which is medically considered to be dangerous to health. Drunkenness among young and underage drinkers is escalating alarmingly, particularly with the advent and seductive marketing of strong 'alco-pop' drinks. People in the 18 to 24 age group are those most likely to commit violent crimes, and are also those most likely to be the victims of violent crime. (Statistics: Social Trends 1996 *Central Statistical Office, United Kingdom.)*

Ready at all times If you have been out for a nice meal with friends, split a few bottles of wine, eaten two puddings, and are basking in the warm glow of a full belly and good conversation, now is the time to remember to be streetwise. If one of your friends is driving you home, or the taxi has been booked, well and good. If you have not made provision for a lift or a taxi, you could be ripe for plucking by local criminals. First of all, book a taxi while you are in the restaurant, asking the management for a reliable firm. If that fails, ring a friend to come and pick you up at the restaurant. It is imperative to avoid a struggle if at all possible, because your reflexes will be slow, and a blow to your full stomach will disable you.

Prostitutes Be especially wary of street girls. It is a fact of life that the areas of cities where the most interesting restaurants can be found are also often areas of high crime rates. In Soho in London, for example, restaurants and brothels exist cheek by jowl. In many old ports throughout the world, the dock areas have become trendy, but also retain a villainous element. 'Honey-pot' muggings, where girls entice a punter to where an accomplice can beat him up and steal his wallet, are commonplace.

Mental attitude

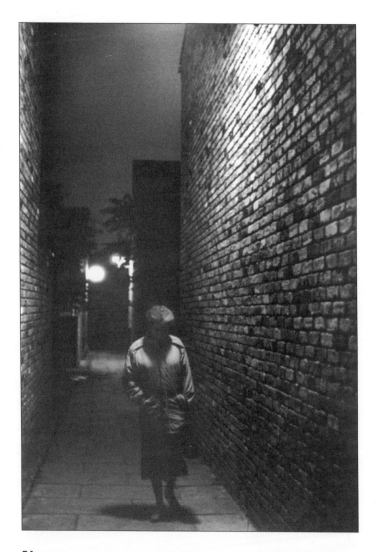

LEFT: Dark alleys and poorly lit streets are to be avoided at all costs, especially if you are alone. Plan your route ahead to avoid potential danger.

Phoning for taxis Use taxis for travelling late at night. You should have the card of a trustworthy firm in your pocket, along with a phone card if you prepared adequately for the evening. Be careful when using a public telephone: it is not unknown for muggers to strike while someone is phoning. Watch the door while you are phoning, and if someone attacks, use the handset as a weapon to hit him in the face if you can. Your best bet is to phone from a pub, and wait there to be collected. When your taxi comes to collect you, make sure it is the one you called, and not a pirate. When you get home have your front door key in your hand.so that you do not have to search your pockets for it. You could also ask the taxi driver to wait until you have entered the house before driving away.

TRAVELLING ON PUBLIC TRANSPORT
Buses are usually fine from the security point of view during the day, as long as they are fairly full of other passengers, but you need to stay alert late in the evening, particularly if there are few other passengers. If the bus is a double decker, it would be foolish to go upstairs and sit at the back, which is about as far away from the driver as it is possible to get. Since the introduction of driver-only buses, the role of the conductor has virtually disappeared. Bus companies save money on wages that way, but the security of passengers is significantly reduced in the process. One security improvement is that on most buses now the driver is in radio contact with inspectors, other drivers and the depot. The sensible rule is to make sure that you are never isolated. Stay downstairs, near the door and among the other passengers. Be where you can attract the attention of the driver if need be.

Late night buses These can be problematic if they are on routes which pick up a lot of young drinkers. So if it is late and you are not confident about the idea of getting the bus, arrange for a lift, or else book a taxi. That way you do not have to wait on the street at the bus stop. If in a group, get a taxi rather than the bus. Stick together as a group, and you are going to be safer. You can drop your friends off one at a time at their homes, and you can share the fare.

Mental attitude

TAXIS

Taxis are not a way round all security problems because not all of them are bona fide. When you hail a taxi in the street, you have no guarantees that the driver is a registered driver working for a reputable firm. There have been cases of drivers posing as cabbies and then raping women they have picked up. Take nothing at face value, including the lighted sign on the roof. Anyone could rig up one of those. The majority of unregistered pirate cab drivers are probably in it to make a bit of money rather than to sexually assault passengers, but you cannot afford to take the risk.

Booking a cab The safest procedure is to book well in advance from a cab firm you know and trust. Ask the controller for the name and number of the driver, and the time it will arrive to pick you up. When the cab arrives, the driver will ask for you by name, and you will know everything is fine. Check his credentials if you are still not sure. Do not enter a taxi if you cannot be certain it is the one you booked. Book the ride from door to door, and you can relax in the knowledge that you do not have to expose yourself to the night streets. If you are caught in a situation where you have to get a ride in the street, take one from a taxi rank rather than hailing a vehicle which is on the move.

Pirate taxis The problems begin to arise when it is late at night, the street is full of people milling around trying to intercept a taxi, and it has started to pour with rain. This is when the pirate drivers are in their element, and people's sense of security flies out of the window. Everything seems to be in short supply, so you grab the first vehicle that slows down. The unlicensed drivers cruise areas which could provide passengers late at night, such as bus stations and train stations. They know the arrival times of late buses and trains, and wait around until the registered cabs have all been taken and driven away before pulling into the ranks to pick up the remaining travellers.

Unlicensed drivers are often spotted and arrested at airports, but no such controls exist at many train stations and bus stations. It pays to cultivate a particular cab firm in you area. Get to know them and their drivers personally, and use them in preference to others. They will appreciate your custom and the custom you can bring them. For your part, it is one less thing to worry about.

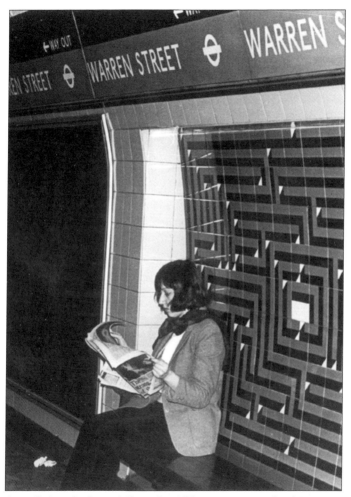

ABOVE: Train and subway stations attract thieves, muggers and rapists, especially at night. Avoid having to wait in such places at night or on your own.

Mental attitude

TRAINS

Trains present similar strategic problems to buses for the solitary traveller, but are potentially more dangerous. Some still have individual carriages rather than through carriages linked by corridors. If you make a mistake you could be stuck in the carriage with undesirable travelling companions long enough to suffer real harm. The dangers begin when you have to wait for a train on a deserted platform.

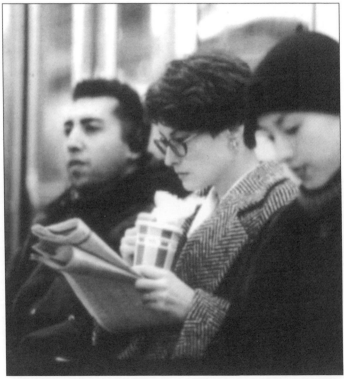

ABOVE: When travelling on trains, always be aware of your fellow passengers even if you are reading. Try to avoid being the only one in a carriage.

Railway stations Away from main stations, many smaller stations are unmanned and poorly lit. Main stations are also dangerous, and attract a variety of criminals, including thieves, pickpockets, muggers, sexual predators and those who prey on young runaways.

Rather than having to spend hours on a station platform or concourse if you miss your train, arrange in advance to stay with trustworthy friends for the night if you have to. Have their phone numbers and a phone card or change with you, and have them come to pick you up in their vehicle or in a cab that they have hired. Contingency planning is the name of the game.

Train carriages If you do catch a train, exercise the same caution you would on a late night bus. Sit where there are several other passengers, including women if you are a woman. Avoid empty compartments, or compartments with one other passenger. There is usually safety in numbers. If someone starts to bother you, move away, and voice your protests loudly if he persists. Be assertive, and remember the disciplines you have practised. If an inspector or guard is available, complain to him. If what appeared to be an innocuous conversation suddenly becomes suggestive, break it off.

Never take anyone at face value, however charming he may seem. Play your hunches. If you have an uncomfortable feeling about someone, however vague, distance yourself from him. The other person might be totally innocent, but until he is proven innocent, you must assume the worst when you are in a vulnerable position. This is not needless paranoia. Intuition has often proved to be justified.

Walking home One problem with stations at night is that if you are leaving them, and there are no taxis, you might have to walk a fair distance to where you can get one. This is probably more dangerous for a woman than for a man. If that happens, all the usual rules apply. If the street is deserted or dark, and you think you are being followed, cross over and head in the opposite direction to make the follower show his hand. If other people are about, you could stop a couple of times to see what the follower does, but do not stop if you are on your own. Do not isolate yourself by running down alleys that may be cul de sacs. If you are on a main street in a town centre, go somewhere that is populated. Look back so that the follower knows that you have

---

Travelling Emergency Equipment

Car maintenance gear should include basic tools, spare sets of plugs, and points, a foot pump, a large bottle of water, and extra fuel in an authorised container It is also a good idea to carry a few things that can increase your security and comfort. A hefty rubberised torch could deter an attacker, as well as being useful if you have to get out and walk to a phone in the dark. Keep a pack of spare batteries with you. A mobile phone is useful wherever you are, to call emergency services to a breakdown, and the police if you are under threat. If you have to look under the bonnet, carry an inspection lamp that can be connected to your car battery, or else use one of the hiking and potholing lamps that you can wear on your head. A large flask of coffee can buoy your spirits and help keep you warm if you have to wait somewhere for a long time, and on a long trip can help you stay awake. Keep a warm blanket or a sleeping bag in the car. A folding shovel can help you dig your way out of snow, or be used to shovel gravel and sand under wheels spinning on ice.

---

noticed him. Think in terms of safe havens – cafés or bars, groups of people around takeaway food shops. Then, if something happens further along the way, you can always retrace your steps to them if you get the chance.

TRAVELLING IN YOUR CAR

When you are travelling alone in your car, there are a number of measures you can take to increase your security. Being in the car gives you a greater measure of protection than if you were walking, but you are not totally immune to the outside world. When you are preparing to set out from your house you are at Level One again. You get your maps out and plan your route. Before doing this you should also, on a regular basis, have gone through routines that ensure the petrol tank is always topped up after using the car, and that the car has been serviced and is reliable.

Fuel Keeping a car topped up is important. Stop to refuel whenever the tank is half empty. If you let the level run right down to near the empty mark, there is a danger of the petrol pump sucking up dregs and dirty fuel from the bottom of the tank, which could cause a blockage and a breakdown. This will inevitably happen, as such things do, when you have to use the car in an emergency in the middle of the night. So fill the tank up as an automatic routine. If you come back exhausted from a long journey, it is easy to leave it until the morning, but then there will be another emergency in the middle of the night, and the clogged fuel pump or whatever will bring you rolling to a halt in the middle of nowhere.

Time management When you are alert and on your guard all the time, the breakdowns do not happen, because you have remembered to fill up the tank and your last service was on time. In an emergency, when you are under pressure, security can tend to evaporate. You leave the house forgetting to lock the doors because you are late, and that is when you get burgled. You take a short cut across some wasteland and are mugged. So always give yourself time. Good time management is as important as a tank full of petrol. Both can save your skin.

Prior planning When you have worked out your route, left a note explaining where you are going, packed your road map and checked for fuel, it is time to leave the house. This is where you go up to Level Two. If the car is in your locked garage there should be no problems, but if it is parked outside, always approach it obliquely at an angle of about 45 degrees. That way you will have a better chance of seeing anyone lurking behind it. Get down briefly and look underneath in order to see the feet of anyone hiding on the other side. You will also see if there are any problems such as a dangling exhaust pipe. Check the back seat before getting in, then get in and lock the doors.

On the road If you are going a long distance, it is a good idea to have a companion who can share the driving – which also makes sense from a security point of view. Stick to the route you have planned out. If you have a mobile phone carry it with you in the car, but keep it with you if you have to get out. If you break down on a motorway, the mobile phone can save you having to walk in the dark and the rain to the next emergency phone as long as you have the phone number of one of the emergency services, and can describe your approximate position. The police advice for those who break down on a motorway is to stay in the car to await the emergency services, but some people prefer to wait up on the bank in case the car is rear-ended by a wandering truck. However, most people stay in the car, and it makes sense for a woman on her own to do so. Put the hazard lights and the interior lights on to make the car more visible.

DRIVING STRATEGIES

It pays to drive defensively in towns and cities. When you you come up to traffic lights at crossroads and T-junctions, position yourself towards the middle of the road, so that you have an option of directions if problems suddenly arise. There is an increasing amount of robbery from cars at traffic lights. Even with the doors locked, a thief may smash a window to grab a briefcase or a mobile phone left on the passenger seat. Always have your window wound up at lights. Keep vulnerable items locked in the boot or under the seats out of sight.

Driving space In traffic, do not drive close up to the car in front or else you may get boxed in by a car coming close up behind you. Maintain enough distance to allow you to go round the car in front if you have to. Be aware of escape routes even when you are in a car. You can use the car to control what happens. By pulling out you can stop someone overtaking you in an emergency security situation. Do not let another car come alongside you to take up the position between you and the kerb in such situations, and in single-line traffic do not get so close to the kerb yourself that a following car can draw alongside you on the outside. Give yourself space all the time.

Breakdowns If you break down and someone walks across offering to give you a hand, you have to use your judgement about their motivations, but keep the doors locked and talk to them through the closed window until you are sure they are genuine. Similarly, if you see someone who has broken down, ask them if they need a hand, but do not impose your assistance on them as they may take it the wrong way and panic. You could tell them that you will call the police for them if they want. A good idea could be to have a few cardboard signs lettered with messages, such as RUN OUT OF PETROL, PLEASE PHONE THE POLICE or I NEED A TOW, which you can put in your window.

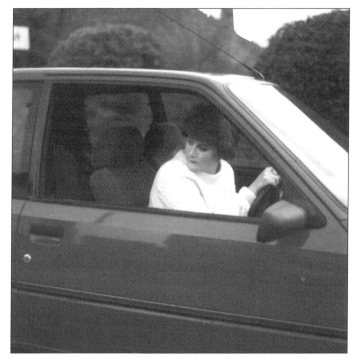

ABOVE: Though you are safer in your car than walking on the street, you still need to be aware of the threats you will face when behind the wheel.

Road rage This is a growing phenomenon which could be connected to the fact that there are now far more cars than ever before, and far more frustration on clogged roads. Avoiding it is partly a matter of making sure you do not do something provocative like cutting someone up or overtaking needlessly. If you do something wrong on the road, like pulling out in front of another car, and the car behind starts flashing its lights, the worst thing you can do is to ignore your mistake and try to speed away. Just stop and say you are sorry, without unlocking the door or opening the window. Acknowledge your mistake in mime. Slap

Miami Car Muggings

Some of the worst cases of car robbery have taken place in Miami in Florida, where a large number of flights arrive carrying European holiday makers. The robbers are completely ruthless, and have killed several of their victims. Their technique is to look for cars bearing the special registration plates of car hire companies which rent to newly arrived air passengers. Miami is notoriously difficult to navigate without local knowledge, and many tourists fresh off the plane lose their way, take wrong turnings, and end up on lonely stretches of motorway. The robbers, who have followed them, or else noticed them trying to read a road map, pull up in front of their victims, sometimes using two cars so that they can box the tourist in. They brandish firearms and demand all money and luggage. Any resistance is met with extreme brutality, and several deaths have occurred in recent years. The car hire companies have taken to using non-identifiable registration plates, but tourists still get lost and drive into danger.

yourself on the wrist. Smile. That way you are showing no aggression, and are defusing the situation. It cannot be misinterpreted, and if they want to take things further, that is their fault.

Even when other cars are in the wrong, do not start tooting your horn. That is calculated to inflame the rage of someone who has had a hard day. If someone blows a horn at you, let it go, even if he is in the wrong. Apologise and smile. Do not be in too much of a hurry to drive off. You do not want to start a race. If you have a powerful and expensive car, do not rise to the bait of inferior cars trying to test you out. Do not race with the battered Mini revving up close behind you. It has probably been stolen, has no insurance, and the driver has nothing to lose by running into the back of you. So swallow any false pride, and do not antagonise him.

Male aggressors Young males sometimes make a game of harassing women in cars, flashing their lights and pretending there is something visibly wrong with the woman's car. Sometimes this is not a game, but a ploy to make her stop, so that she can be mugged. If your car feels all right to drive, be very reluctant to stop. Continue driving until you come to a well lit place such as a garage, where you can get help. Do not stop in a lonely place. If you think the car flashing you might be someone in authority, pull over but keep your engine running. If it is not the police, and they get out of their car and come towards you, drive away. Always try to have an escape route.

DISTRACTION TECHNIQUES

If you have to leave your vehicle for any reason and are pursued by an attacker, you must try to gain time. To do this, try distracting your opponent. Some distraction techniques have been described above, but one of the most effective can be used once the confrontation is inevitable. When boxers throw a punch, they try to get all the air out of the body as they do so. They exhale vigorously with each punch, and the effect is to tighten up the diaphragm. In that way they are not winded if they take a counter punch in the stomach or solar plexus. A similar technique is used in martial arts to focus all the energy into a strike, sometimes accompanied by a yell. By breathing out forcibly and striking, you get maximum power. In a real life confrontation, you can use the same technique. Make your mind up without signalling your intentions, and then suddenly let loose with a great scream, 'YEEEEAAH!' Get rid of all your inhibitions, and spit all over the guy as you launch yourself forward. This will drive him back onto his rear foot. Once he starts going backwards you are in control. You just keep steaming forward without giving him a chance as you drive home the combination strikes you have been practising.

The element of surprise The essence of success is surprise in this and most other self-defence techniques. Surprise has to be backed up with all the commitment and training that this book tries to instil. To survive in the modern world we cannot afford to have a passive outlook. We would all like a peaceful life, but we have to be prepared for anything to happen. People think it will never happen to them, but it does, with depressing frequency.

Training your body and your mind for self-defence is a good investment. This is not to say you should live your life with a siege mentality, far from it, but it is prudent to be prepared for the worst. Even if nothing ever happens to you, you will have immeasurably improved the quality of your life.

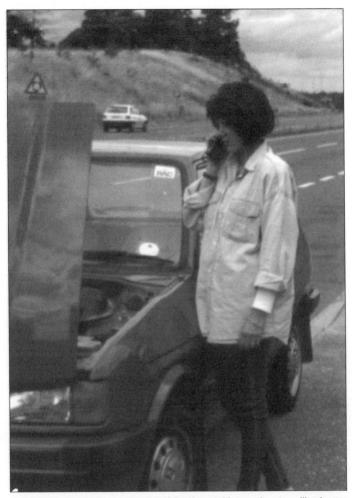

ABOVE: It is a good idea to carry a mobile phone with you when travelling by car. If you break down, it will save you having to walk to emergency telephones.

SELF-DEFENCE TECHNIQUES

The advice and self-defence moves which are presented in the following pages are the result of years of experience. They are a blend of different martial arts styles, and are designed to enable someone being attacked to successfully defend themself and escape in the minimum amount of time. They are the techniques used by the **SAS**, amended for civilian use.

CHAPTER 1
LEARNING SELF-DEFENCE

There is no substitute for joining a local martial arts club and practising self-defence moves on a regular basis. It does not matter what style you choose, just get yourself along to a club and before long the blocks, strikes and throws will become second nature.

To learn how to defend yourself, you really need to practise. Books, films and videos are all useful, but don't come anywhere near regular practice. I would advise anyone to take up a martial art, and not just for self-defence reasons. Although a lot of martial arts skills are not directly applicable to self-defence, training in any art gives you confidence and improves your speed, timing and balance, These benefits are also useful for normal daily life, as is the self-discipline you gain from such training. And this discipline is especially valuable to young people, and can contribute to them keeping out of trouble themselves.

What style? No one martial art is good for all situations. Each art or style concentrates on different elements, and most have sporting applications, and thus have rules. Grappling arts, such as judo, usually

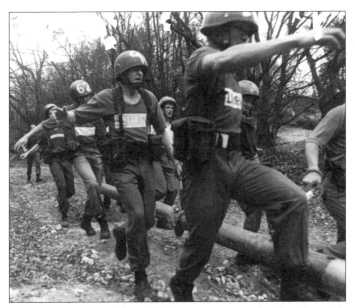

Above: As well as practising self-defence moves, you should endeavour to improve your general fitness. Greater fitness will improve your reaction times.

depend on an attacker wearing a loose jacket such as a judo uniform, and can be less effective if he is wearing a tight T-shirt or no shirt at all. All arts have limitations, whether due to sporting rules or the restraints of safe practice. This book takes bits from all sorts of martial arts, and blends them with the fruits of hard experience.

But any martial art taught by a good instructor is useful and forms a good sound basis for building on. I recommend that you take up the one that suits you best. Your build, suppleness, fitness, agility, age and mental condition all influence the best style of fighting for you. If you are tall, you have the reach to box, and can keep people away from you. Shorter people need to be able to duck and weave to come inside an attacker's reach. If you are big and powerful, you can grab hold of people and put locks on them. But whatever style you prefer, you have

Self-defence techniques

to be able to adapt it to the situation you are in, so the more styles and the more knowledge you've got, the better equipped you are.

If you ever have to use self-defence techniques in a real situation, you are going to be scared and under a lot of pressure. So it's got to be a fast and natural reaction. You need to be able to adapt without thinking, so that if you, say, miss with a kick, you don't stop, but rather switch into another technique.

Practice Put as much time into learning self-defence techniques as you can. If it's only one hour a month that's better than nothing. Once you get into a training discipline, its a healthier way of life and you feel better, more confident. If you join a club and you don't like it, leave it. Do something else. There are some very good instructors, but unfortunately there are also bad ones, so ideally you should pick one who is recommended and who is acknowledged to be good. Keep it up.

You can also get useful practice outside the confines of the martial arts club. You can hang a punch bag and practise on that. You can also practise at home (safely!) with a friend or partner. Get them to 'attack' you in different ways, and practise what you have learnt in your training class. If you can practise with someone else in your class, you can both benefit. The ideal is to train with as many different people as possible. In most training situations, everyone starts by training with friends. You soon get used to this, so you should switch around as much as possible. You end up faced with people of differing heights, weights, age and strength, so your reactions don't become stereotyped. You can't pick an aggressor out there, he is going to pick you. So don't get set in your ways, and make sure you keep on changing training partners.

Mental training You should also practise mentally. You can go over the basics in your mind, even while waiting for a bus. You can also 'play through' different situations, trying to analyse potential threats and working out how you would deal with them. When I am working on a security job, I do a lot of travelling, and spend hours at airports. Rather than waste this time, I play mind games with myself. I look around anywhere, any room, and work out where the safest place to be is. For instance, I avoid plate glass windows, because if there's a bomb blast they can break, chandeliers can come down, walls collapse and so on. At a simpler level, rubbish bins may harbour bees, wasps and hornets, so I look around, check out the environment, thinking, 'Ah, if I sit in that corner there, and I watch this and I watch that, then I'm safe.' I also look around at other people, analysing them and their actions. Is he a member of security? Is he thinking like me? I am looking for escape routes, or deciding who is the most likely threat here. For instance, the man over there has a large suitcase – what's in it? Or that workman over there has a chisel – if I'm attacked, where's the best escape route? So all the time I am aware of what's going on around me, and working out the best reaction to any danger.

Mental agility You don't need to be a security professional to benefit from mental training like this. And while you don't want to bring on paranoia, you can do similar exercises in daily life. For instance, I may be standing at a bus stop. Who's behind me? What are they carrying? If I have to run, where is the best direction? Look upon these exercises as being fun and a challenge – they will stand you in good stead in a self-defence situation

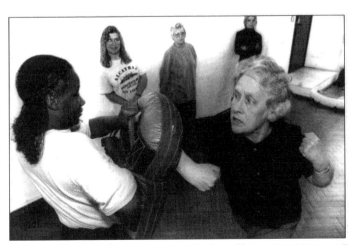

ABOVE: Self-defence is for everyone, no matter how old or young or big or small you are. Choose a particular style which suits you, and stick at it.

CHAPTER 2

YOUR BODY'S WEAPONS

Most parts of the body, if used correctly, can be used to defend yourself from an attacker. You may think you are unarmed, but the reality is that with the proper training and knowledge you can call upon your own personal arsenal to beat off and escape from violent assaults.

For most people, the only weapons they will have to hand in a self-defence situation will be their limbs. When used correctly, they can be extremely effective, allowing you to defeat an attack and escape. This chapter shows what your body's weapons are, and how they should be used in self-defence.

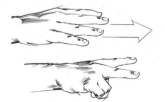

When using the fingers to jab, use all four (top). The two-fingered jab (bottom) has less chance of connecting with the target.

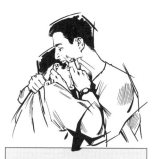

The teeth can be very useful in self-defence. If you're a woman, bite on whatever you can get hold of, ideally the ear. And once you bite don't let go – you'll just arouse the attacker. Bite into his neck, his throat, his ear; just bite, chew, rip and spit.

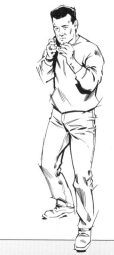

Fighting stance: knees slightly bent, chin down, elbows in and hands up.

THE CORRECT STANCE

If trouble is about to start and you can't get away quickly, you need to be in a stable stance: one that is well balanced but allows you to move easily in any direction. Keep your feet about shoulder width apart, no more than 45cm (18in), with your weight evenly balanced across both of them. Try to stand at an oblique angle to a potential attacker, say some 30 degrees or so. I prefer to stand with my left leg slightly forward; some prefer to go the other way, but I would say if in doubt put your left leg forward. This gives you good balance front and back, as well as to either side.

Stand on the balls of your feet so you have your weight and centre of balance in the middle. Keep your knees slightly bent, your chin down, elbows in to your side and your hands up. Don't form a fist:

Self-defence techniques

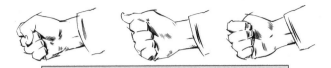

To form a fist, curl the fingers in against the palm and tuck your thumb down the outside (left). Don't tuck the thumb inside your fingers (right), or rest it on your forefinger (centre).

you have much more flexibility with your hands open. Also, this is not an overtly aggressive stance, but standing with your fists clenched like a boxer signals an intention to stand and fight, and may trigger a situation you can still avoid.

Whatever stance you choose, stick to it. You need to feel comfortable and secure with whatever stance you choose. Even most professional fighters don't change stances from left to right, they stick to one and master it.

THE HEAD

Your body comes complete with a host of natural weapons. Starting at the top, there is your head. This is a big, bony structure. The hardest part of the skull is the back, while the forehead and bone structure around the face is also fairly strong. For a smaller person grabbed by someone larger, the head can be a devastating weapon. You can use your forehead to butt him anywhere in the face. If you hit above the eyes this will probably cause a cut, and although he should be able to see through the blood, many people go to pieces once they know they are bleeding. You need to keep your chin tucked in to protect your neck, and make sure you don't bite your tongue! If you are held in a tight grip and can't move your arms or knees, the head butt is a good opener to make him let go. It can also be effective if you are grabbed from behind. You just snap your head back into him, shoving the hard part of your head straight backwards into his face.

You have to bear in mind though that the top of your head is vulnerable, and a strike to that part or the temples can be extremely dangerous for the victim. You should never strike someone in the temples unless your life is at risk.

Teeth The head is also where the teeth are located. No matter how weak or unfit you are, a bite can cause an incredible amount of pain if an attacker gets within range. This can be especially useful for women, for if an assault has a sexual motive, the attacker's ear, or sometimes hands, are going to be within reach of your mouth. When a dog bites, it doesn't have that much power, but what it does is bite, hang on and rip and tear. Then at least in a line-up when there's a suspect with one ear missing, you can say, 'Yes, that guy tried to rape me, because here's his ear.'

HANDS

Most people think of using the hands to punch an attacker, but I don't recommend that. It takes a lot of training to develop a hard, accurate punch, and without this you are more likely to hurt your own hand without doing a great deal of damage. But what you can do is strike with the fingers.

If someone is coming in towards you, the most effective strike is a jab with your fingers into the eyes. Go straight for the eyes and use all

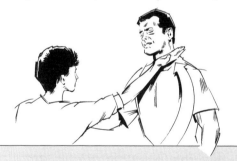

The side of the hand can be used to strike an attacker's soft areas, such as the throat or side of the neck. Keep the fingers straight and hit with the fleshy edge of the hand.

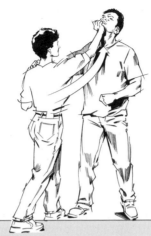

Executing a palm strike: your palm is drawn back and then you drive it up and forward. Twist your body into it, and try to step forward as you strike to put your weight behind the blow.

your fingers extended in a fast snapping strike. Don't just use two fingers, that's mainly for films. All your fingers should be extended, but not locked straight: you should have them in a very slight curve so that if you miss and hit bone, you don't break them. With all four fingers extended, your chance of an accurate strike is much better, and even if you only get one eye, the pain will distract your attacker, and possibly even cause him to lose his balance. This won't necessarily win the fight straight away, but it does open an attacker up to further moves.

Your fingers are also essential for grappling and for applying various locks to the attacker's wrists and fingers (see Chapter 5).

Palm strikes The hand is also used for striking, and I recommend that you use the palm of the hand. If an attacker is in front of you, you can step forward and strike with the heel of the palm up into his chin. It takes a lot less skill than a punch, it won't damage your hand, and

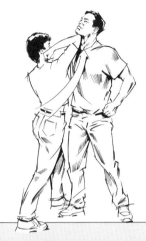

The elbows are powerful weapons. If an attacker is in front of you, for example, you can swing your elbow up and into his face. Don't forget to throw your weight into the strike.

can be much more devastating. It is best if combined with an earlier distraction strike, ideally the fingers to the eyes as described above. It's not a jab, it's a full-blooded strike. Come in towards your opponent as you hit and follow through past the point of impact. Drive the palm up into his chin – if you miss you can continue the move into his nose.

Punches A punch may be useful if you are against someone whom you do not want to hurt, such as an annoying drunk. Here you can dig him in the stomach with a punch. The first thing is to form the fist properly. Curl the fingers in tightly against the palm, and tuck your thumb down the outside, across the index and middle fingers. Don't tuck the thumb inside your fingers, and don't have it resting on the top of your forefinger. When you throw a punch, you need to line up the bones and muscles in your arm, and you should twist your arm as you throw the punch, so that you hit with your palm down. The top knuckles

Self-defence techniques

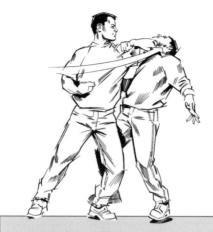

With a side elbow strike, bring your arm across the front of your chest, palm inwards, then thrust back along the same route, driving the the elbow into the attacker's face or throat.

should be in line with the wrist, and the main impact should be with the first and second knuckles.

But to get force behind a punch, you need to get your body into it. Twist forward from the waist as the arm moves, and before your arm is fully extended. The energy should come from your hips and waist, not just the shoulders. Don't expect to win a fight with the first punch either – even an experienced boxer doesn't try for that. Use the first punch or two to distract an opponent; open him up by making him block your attacks before you step in with one or two finishing strikes.

The chop The side of the hand can also be used to hit an opponent, especially against soft areas like the throat or side of the neck. This is also a good way to attack joints such as the inside of the elbow, which will help to loosen an attacker's grip. Keep the fingers straight and hit with the fleshy edge between the wrist and the base of the fingers.

ELBOWS

Everyone has elbows, and they are always hard, bony and pointed. They make excellent weapons at close range, delivering a surprising amount of power without requiring a great degree of skill to use.

KNEES

Your legs have some of the most powerful muscles in your body, and the bony knee can deliver incredibly effective strikes at close range. If you are comparatively light or small, you can still deliver a powerful blow without too much effort. For instance, if you are a woman being harassed by a drunk at a party, after telling him to go away, you can possibly drive your knee into the side of his thigh, halfway between the hip and the knee. This is the 'dead leg'. It won't do any real damage, but it can temporarily paralyse the muscles, causing him to fall over. Then you can walk away quickly.

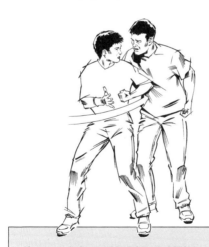

If you are being grabbed from behind, you can twist and drive your elbow back into the stomach. Combine this with a short step to the outside, which opens up his body as a target.

Self-defence techniques

Dead leg

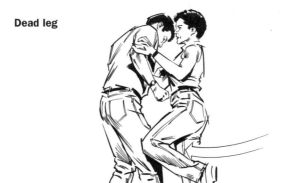

The knees can be very effective weapons. This is the dead leg, which involves driving the knee into the side of an attacker's thigh, halfway between the hip and knee.

If the threat is more menacing, the same knee hard into the groin will put your attacker out of action for longer, and allow you to get well clear before he can even think about moving. If it doesn't work first time, grab on and keep striking, and if he doubles up, grab his head and smash your knee into his face.

FEET
A skilled martial artist can kick a door off its hinges, but you won't see many trying such techniques in a real situation. The only kick I would consider using is a side kick. Here, if you turn side on to an opponent, you can thrust out with the sole of the foot. Keep the kick low, preferably at his knees, and bring your foot back fast. The advantage of this kick is that you don't risk losing your balance if you miss.

Side kick

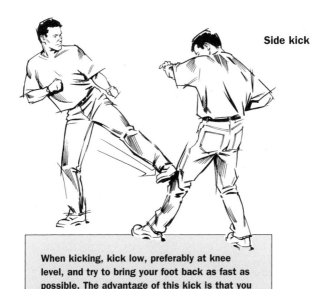

When kicking, kick low, preferably at knee level, and try to bring your foot back as fast as possible. The advantage of this kick is that you don't risk losing your balance if you miss.

If an attacker is standing very close to you, short stamping kicks to his knees, legs, ankles or feet can be useful. If he is facing you, you can stamp down onto his knee. This can damage his kneecap, and even if you miss, your foot will rake down his shin and onto his instep. If he is side-on to you, a sideways stamp to the knee has a chance of breaking the knee joint. If he is grappling you from behind, a stamping kick backwards can hurt his shin.

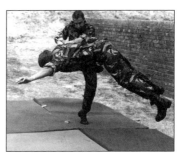

ABOVE: When using kicks in a self-defence situation remember to keep them low and simple. Fancy techniques are for the experts.

CHAPTER 3

EVERYDAY ITEMS IN SELF-DEFENCE

Innocuous items such as newspapers and walking sticks can be potential life-savers in a self-defence situation, giving you extra aids with which to fend off an attacker.

I wouldn't recommend that anyone carry a weapon. Guns, knives, chemical sprays, electric stunners are all illegal in most countries, and could get you into more trouble with the law than you would have been with the original attack. I think that carrying a weapon, such as a knife, takes you over the line between being a person defending yourself, and someone who is looking for trouble. You might do terrible damage to someone who doesn't necessarily deserve it. The same applies to some of the more destructive everyday implements that may be to hand, such as a beer glass, screwdriver or hammer. In addition, most people don't actually have the will to use a dangerous weapon. Unless you are determined, waving a knife at someone might just give them the opportunity to take it away and use it against you. And finally, the fact that you are carrying a weapon may give you a false, undeserved

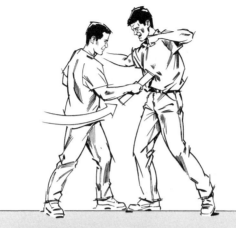

A rolled-up newspaper can be used to devastating effect against an attacker. Driven into the stomach, for example, it will wind an opponent, allowing you to escape.

sense of security. With all personal security, the aim is to avoid trouble, not to go out to meet it head on. That said, there are many everyday objects that can be pressed into service in an emergency. The first one to look at is a specialised, relatively inoffensive martial arts tool which usually doubles as a large keyholder.

The 'Kubotan' This is a short bar, some 15cm (6in) long and 1cm (.5in) in diameter, made from hard plastic or aluminium, with big ribs on it and a rounded tapered point at one end. It usually has a hole at the other end, allowing it to hold your keys. This can be used in various ways to inflict pain on an attacker without being particularly dangerous to them. If you don't have a Kubotan, any hard bar shape, such as a ball-point pen, can make a useful substitute

If someone grabs you, for instance by grasping your shirt or jacket, you can lie the Kubotan across the nerve at the top of the wrist. Hold

Self-defence techniques

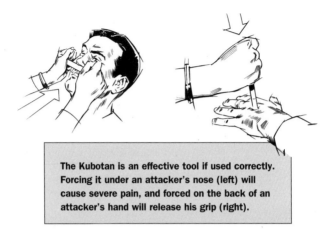

The Kubotan is an effective tool if used correctly.
Forcing it under an attacker's nose (left) will
cause severe pain, and forced on the back of an
attacker's hand will release his grip (right).

both ends of the Kubotan, then roll it downwards and into your chest. This will inflict pain on the wrist and should cause the attacker to drop down into a crouch. You can then drive your knee into his face before escaping. Pushing the Kubotan hard between his fingers, squeezing them tightly together, will also cause a fair amount of pain.

The Kubotan can also be used as a jabbing weapon by driving it into soft areas on your attacker's body. For instance, if someone places their hand on your thigh, you can jab down hard onto the back of his hand with the Kubotan. The space between the bone structure that forms the root of the middle and ring fingers is best. You can also use this defence if someone has grabbed your hand and is trying to drag you along. If you haven't got a weapon to hand, drive your thumb hard into the same spot and keep working hard on it until he lets go. But a pen, the handle of a hairbrush, or any pointed, hard object, will do.

If someone is facing you and coming towards you, you can drive the Kubotan into the soft area of the neck below the Adam's apple and above the 'v' made by the clavicle bones. Push hard, which will make an attacker step back and let go of you. If he has a tight hold, such as a bear hug, from the front, hold it horizontally, with one hand on either end, and drive it side-on, hard up into the base of his nose, pushing his head up and back until he lets go. Another target is in the

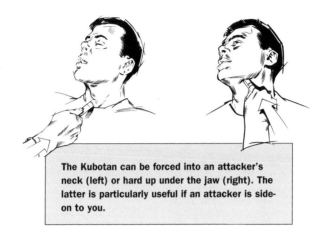

The Kubotan can be forced into an attacker's neck (left) or hard up under the jaw (right). The latter is particularly useful if an attacker is side-on to you.

soft area under the jaw, directly in line with the ear. Swing the pen or Kubotan around the side and drive hard up under the jaw. This is useful if someone is side-on to you – for instance, if an attacker is alongside you in your car.

If he is further away, an alternative target is the soft area on the shoulder. Jabbing the Kubotan into the gap between the collar bone and the shoulder join, can often force an attacker to drop that arm back away from you. If nothing else, you can grip the Kubotan in your hand to make a punch heavier, more effective and safer for your hands. Any other small heavy object can help here.

Walking sticks The Kubotan, while not an offensive weapon, is still something that you have to decide to carry in advance of any threat. But what about improvised weapons that come to hand? If you walk with a stick or cane, this can be used to protect you from an attack. Hold the stick in two hands, with the hand at the front palm upwards and the hand at the back palm down. Leave some stick protruding at both ends. You can use it to deflect punches or kicks, to block knife or glass attacks, or to strike or jab an assailant. The worst thing you can do is swing it like a sword, as an attacker with any speed can get inside your swing and take the stick from you. Some martial art styles

Self-defence techniques

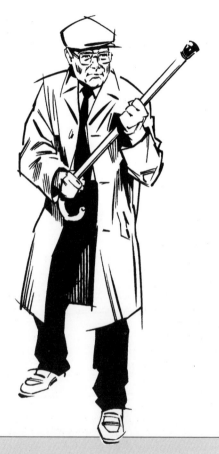

A walking stick can be a useful self-defence aid.
Hold it like a quarter staff for jabs and blocks.
Do not start swinging it like a sword, as an
attacker might catch it and yank it away.

specialise in using sticks to lock up elbows, shoulders or wrists, but these techniques demand a lot of practice.

Sprays and newspapers Other items you might carry normally include hair or deodorant sprays. These are also a useful defence against dangerous dogs. A comb, especially if it is metal, can be raked across someone's face, while something as innocuous as a plastic credit card can be wedged up under the nose. A magazine or newspaper, if rolled up tightly, can be driven into an attacker's stomach or solar plexus. You can also jab it into vulnerable areas like the throat.

Bags If you have a bag or handbag, swing it around hard. It might not make contact, but it will make someone step back. And if you have bags of shopping, why not lift out a tin of beans? It could give you a vital second either to get away or close in and finish him off.

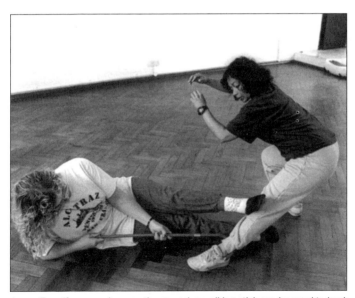

ABOVE: *Even if you are down on the ground, a walking stick can be used to hook an attacker's leg, giving you valuable seconds to get up and escape.*

CHAPTER 4

TARGET AREAS ON THE BODY

Successful self-defence is as much about being able to strike the right target as it is being able to perform the actual moves. A knowledge of an attacker's vulnerable spots is essential if you are going to achieve your aim, which is to defeat him in a matter of seconds.

If you get into a fight or are attacked, there is no point in just flailing away madly, you need to have a target in mind for each blow or grab. So let's look at some of the weak spots on an opponent's body.

THE HEAD
Where the head goes, so does the rest of the body. The best way to put someone on the ground is to push his chin back then turn his head. If he braces his neck, push back first with a palm strike to the chin, then turn his head to one side. You can combine this with jabs to the eyes or strikes under the nose before he goes down.

The eyes The head also holds other vulnerable targets. The eyes are probably the most obvious. A finger jabbed into them, or a comb raked across sideways will cause extreme pain. If you are being grabbed, you can even run your hands up your attacker's face until your fingers find his eyes and then just jab them in. A successful attack will cause extreme pain, while his tear ducts will produce so much water that it will make it nearly impossible for your attacker to see where you are. Jabs to the eyes are also good for opening up an opponent to further attacks. Even if your strike fails to make proper contact, his reflex will be to shut his eyes tightly and try to defend with his hands. He is now wide open for another attack, whether to the head, torso or legs.

The nose The base of the nose and the upper lip have a large number of nerve endings, and can be very painful if pushed or struck. If someone is close, striking or pushing upwards into the base of the nose will cause his head to go back. You can also use the nose as a lever, by driving fingers into his nostrils and pulling or pushing up.

And if someone is trying to bite you, don't pull back, that just helps him cause damage. Instead, push into his mouth, at the same time driving your fingers or thumbs into his cheek. This pushes the flesh into his own teeth, making it impossible for him to bite down hard.

The ears These are a good target for biting, especially if you are a woman and the attack has a sexual nature. His ears will be in just the right place for you to clamp your teeth on to.

But a word of warning. You can easily cause severe or even fatal damage by attacking the head in the wrong way. Never club down on the top of the head, especially with a weapon. Similar warnings apply to the neck and throat. Don't attack the throat, or strike the side of the neck with a weapon, as this could cause unconsciousness and death.

THE TORSO
The central torso is pretty strong, although this depends to some extent on the level of fitness of the attacker. A knee into the stomach can sometimes wind someone, but you shouldn't rely on it. The kidneys are relatively unprotected to the rear, and a blow here can cause extreme pain.

The groin This is extremely vulnerable, in women as well as in men. A knee, a kick, a punch or a strike from the side of a hand can all cause

Self-defence techniques

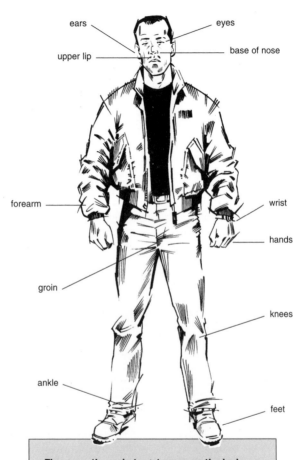

ears

eyes

upper lip

base of nose

forearm

wrist

hands

groin

knees

ankle

feet

These are the main target areas on the body.
Jabs, strikes and stamps against these areas
– especially the eyes and the groin – will
incapacitate an attacker.

great pain. And if you are being held in close, a tight grab can get your opponent's total attention.

ARMS
If you have a stick or club, you can strike the wrist, the top of the forearm, or the inside of the upper arm muscle. A good hit in any of these places will cause pain, and may deaden the limb, or even break the wrist joint. None of them is likely to be permanently harmful, but will allow you to escape an attack.

HANDS
If someone is grabbing you, the hands are an obvious target. The fingers can all be bent back, and this will cause great pain with comparatively little effort. You can also grab one finger in each hand and pull them wide apart for a similar effect. If you can get your hand onto an attacker's thumb, by pushing back you can make him loosen any grip he might have, such as on your arm. His wrist joint can also be used to create locks, by trying to force his hand in a direction in which it would not naturally move.

LEGS
The knees are extremely vulnerable, especially on larger, heavy men. You can stamp down on the front of the kneecap, and if you hit you are going to disconnect it. If you miss, you slide your foot all the way down the shin and thump it onto the foot. A similar stamping attack to the side of the knee can also break it, while stamping into the back of the knee will fold the leg, usually dropping the attacker on the ground.

Another target on the legs is the 'dead leg' area, the nerve point in the side of the thigh, halfway between the hip and knee. The value of this attack, and hitting the nerve points on the arm, is that it will work no matter how psyched up an attacker is.

FEET
You can stamp down on an attacker's foot, and this can be especially effective if you are a woman wearing stiletto heels. If you put your full weight onto someone's foot, it can trap him. From here a firm shove will cause him to loose his balance and fall to the ground. This gives you time either to finish him off or get away.

CHAPTER 5

DEFENCE TECHNIQUES

The self-defence techniques illustrated in the following pages are designed to defeat a variety of attacks. Irrespective of how big or small you are, these techniques will enable you to defend yourself with the minimum of force but with maximum effectiveness.

These self-defence techniques should only be used as a last resort. In any threat scenario keep talking: "Don't do it, don't do it, stay back." Until an attack starts, remain in the ready stance even while being relaxed and non-confrontational. But if a fight starts, you can block, parry, evade, or strike with the hands, elbows or feet. The following self-defence moves combine blocks, strikes and escapes until your attacker is down and out of the fight, or you are able to run away. If you are attacked, you should try to defeat your opponent as quickly as possible. I must stress that you should practise the following techniques until they become second nature, instinctive almost. However, always try to evade violence if you can. Even if you are made to look foolish and a coward, so what, you will still be alive.

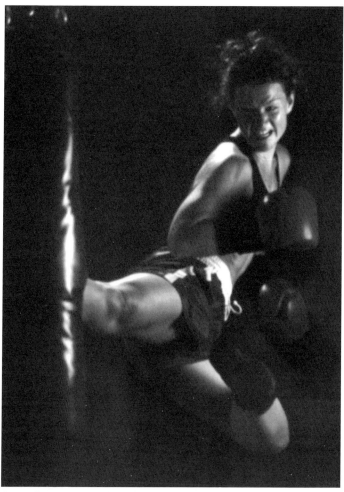

ABOVE: Constant self-defence training will give you the strength, power and confidence to deter most would-be attackers, and deal with them in a fight.

Blocks

Blocks should always be used as a prelude to a counterattack, which should be continued until your attacker is incapable of further assault.

Defence against straight punch

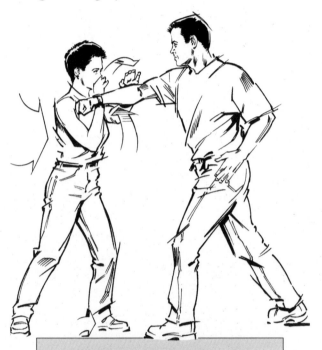

If someone throws a punch, the first thing you have to do is avoid being hit. If it is a straight blow, swing out of the way, while bringing your hand and arm up sharply across your body to deflect the strike.

Follow-up palm strike

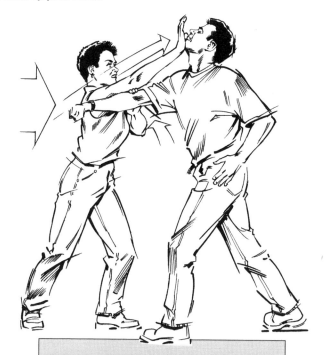

Once you have blocked the punch, and before he has time to recover, a good counter is to step in towards him, twisting from the hips and striking upwards to his chin with the heel of your palm. If you took his balance with the block, this will dump him on his back, probably whacking his head on the ground. Another technique is to step in again, but this time swinging your elbow up and into his chin. Remember to try to keep your own balance at all times.

Self-defence techniques

Blocking a hooked punch

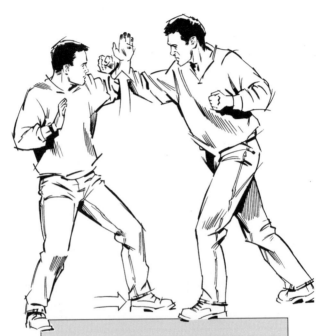

If the punch is hooked or swung around (a 'roundhouse' punch), don't try to step outside the punch – you'll walk right into it if you do. And don't try to keep your distance, it means that you will be meeting the punch just as it reaches its maximum energy. Instead, you should step towards the attacker while blocking, using the hard bony top of your forearms on the inside of his arm. If he has a weapon, you can also block in the same way.

Follow-up palm strike

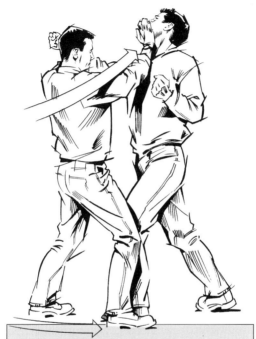

Once you are inside, you are ideally placed for a palm heel to his chin, a finger jab to his eyes, or a combination of both. When executing any strike, be sure to use your body weight to maximum effect. As shown here, after blocking the punch, you should step forward with the right leg and simultaneously thrust the right hip forward to give the palm strike added momentum and power.

Self-defence techniques

Two-handed block against a hooked punch

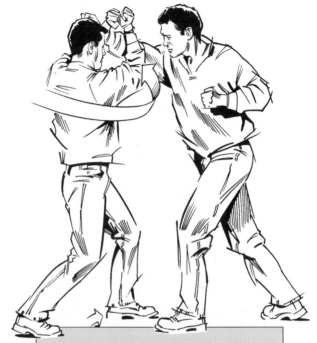

If you are pitted against a tall or very strong attacker, you can use a two-handed block against a hooked punch. Again you must step into the punch to defeat it, although in this case you may want to use both your forearms in the block as shown here. You will then be in a position to deliver a variety of strikes against your attacker's head, though you must carry out your counterattack in a split-second.

Follow-up elbow strike

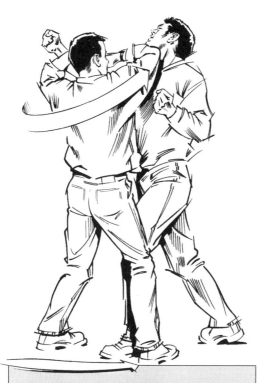

Having performed a two-handed block against a hooked punch (if your attacker has a weapon, you can also block in the same way), you can deliver an elbow strike against his chin, or a finger jab to the eyes, then maybe a backhand to the bridge of the nose. But whatever you do, the strikes must be fast and accurate.

Self-defence techniques

Defence against knee strike

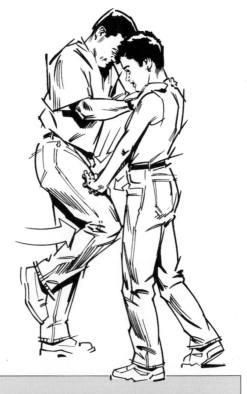

An attacker may try to use his knee against you, for instance by pulling your head down towards his knee. Turn towards the knee that he is using and block down using both hands.

Follow-up elbow strike

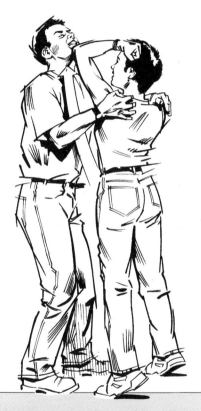

After blocking his knee strike, straighten up, and at the same time come up with an elbow strike through his arms. Then throw a short but heavy punch into his stomach.

Self-defence techniques

Ground defence 1

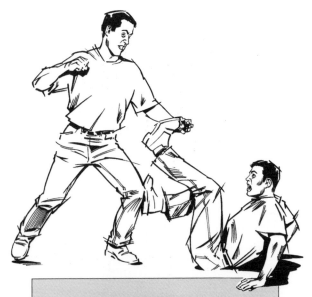

If you have slipped or been knocked down,
you need to keep defending yourself. The most
common attack here is the stamp or kick. If
someone is going to kick you, pivot on your back
so that your feet are towards them. Bend your
legs so that your shins are covering your groin,
then keep flicking your legs out to his in short
sharp kicks. You might catch his legs, while the
continuing movement gives him no clear target.
If he gets close enough, go for a hard kick to his
shin or kneecap, which might take him down if
it connects. Push down with your elbows to get
leverage and increase the force behind the kick.

Ground defence 2

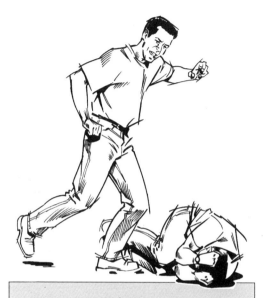

If you can't get into the position illustrated opposite, and a number of attackers are kicking at you while you are on the ground, you need to do what you can to protect your vital organs. So curl up into a ball, with your arms over your head and your knees and shins up protecting your stomach and groin. Do what you can, though, and keep your brain working. For instance, you can try to get against a wall or into the corner of a room to protect your back, or under a table if you are indoors – anything to hamper your attackers. You are very vulnerable when on the ground.

Self-defence techniques

Counterattack from ground 1

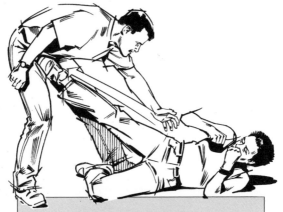

If you cannot get up from the ground for any reason you must fight back hard by aiming blows at the attacker's vital areas. The groin is a good target to aim for. If you are on the ground and an attacker comes in close over you, as if he is about to bend down to strangle or rape you, you can drive up with your heel into his groin. If you are on your side, push down with your elbows to get leverage and increase the force behind the kick. Once again it must be stressed that your priority when on the ground is to get up. The longer you are down the less chance you have of getting back up again. It is therefore imperative to make your attacks count – you will not have the time or energy to put up a prolonged fight from this position. Remember, even an experienced martial artist faces a difficult task if on the ground.

Counterattack from ground 2

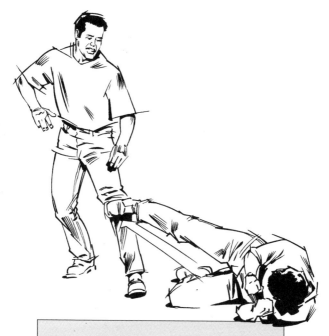

This is a variation of the attack shown on page 104. The shins and knees are excellent targets when fighting from the ground. Remember, lying on your side, be it left or right, allows you to use your arms and legs for support. When you have hit your attacker's knee or shin, get up before he can recover. Never choose to continue fighting from the ground. The reality is that you will probably only have one chance to deliver a strike while on the ground.

Defence against grabs

The following self-defence techniques for escaping various grabs will allow you to break free from an assailant very quickly.

Escape from double wrist grab 1

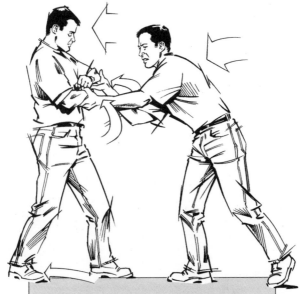

If someone has grabbed your wrists, you need to break out through the weakest part of his grip, through the gap between the fingertips and the thumb. Twist your wrists inwards, until your thumbs are pointing up, then move your hands up and back as you step back. This move can be applied if only one wrist is grabbed, but be aware of the attacker's other hand.

Escape from double wrist grab 2

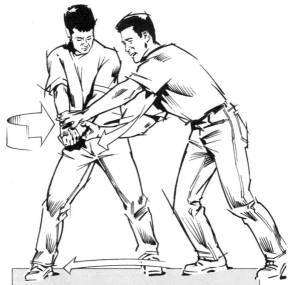

This is an alternative defence against having both wrists grabbed Turn your body as you pull your arms back. This will pull the attacker off balance if he tries to hold on. In such a position he is very vulnerable to a counterattack, though you will have to judge the level of response. If you are a woman, for example, and a drunken man has attempted to grab you in a bar or night club, you may decide that breaking free of his grasp and walking away is enough. If, on the other hand, the grab is a more serious assault, your response may be a palm or elbow strike to the attacker's face.

Self-defence techniques

Defence against front hair grab

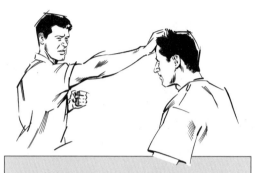

If you have long or bushy hair, you are a prime target for this type of attack, so as soon as an attacker grabs your hair, swing all your weight on the opposite side.

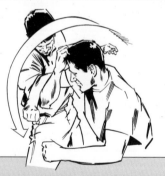

If he grabs you with his right, throw all your weight to your left, and swing your own right arm over his as shown above. This will throw your attacker off-balance.

Elbow strike

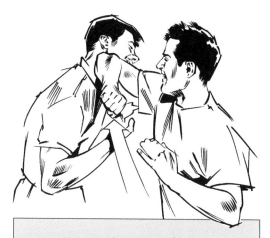

You can usually get a strike in with your elbow
as you do this. You can then snap your elbow
back into the side of his face, which you have
just pulled down into range. Don't forget your
other hand: as your attacker is off-balance and
reeling from your elbow strike, try to deliver
a palm strike under his nose with your other
hand. Or, as your attacker will have undoubtedly
released his grip, a knee to the groin.

Self-defence techniques

Defence against rear hair grab 1

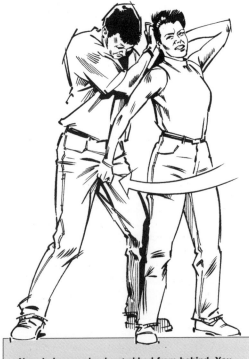

Your hair may also be grabbed from behind. You need to pivot fast into your attacker. Keep your arm and hand straight, and use the edge of the hand to strike into your attacker's groin.

Defence against rear hair grab 2

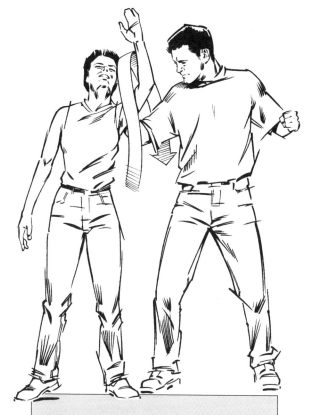

Another defence against a rear hair grab is again to pivot into your attacker, but this time push your arm up and over the top of his. As with all the self-defence techniques illustrated, your reflexes and timing need to be very quick to gain the advantage.

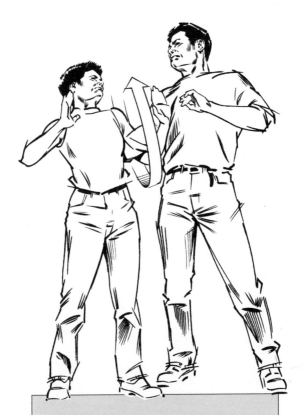

You can wrap your own arm over the attacker's grabbing arm and lock up his arm or elbow as you step in with a palm heel strike to the chin. Locking his arm will also have the effect of forcing his body to the rear and off-balance. This will give you time to decide what strike you want to execute.

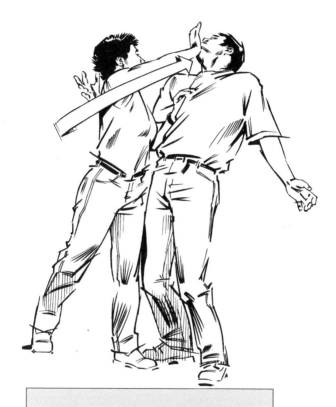

You can use an elbow strike instead of a palm strike if you are close enough, but you must get at least one strike in to get him to release you. You could try a knee strike to the groin.

Self-defence techniques

Defence against simultaneous grab and punch

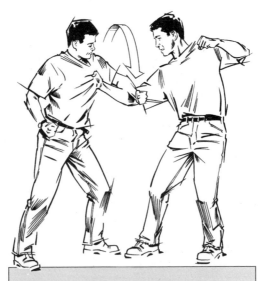

A common attack, especially in a bar, is for
someone to grab your clothing with one hand
and line up a punch with the other. In this
case, the attacker is grabbing with the right in
preparation for a punch with his left hand. As
the grab and punch usually follow each other
quickly, you must immediately twist slightly to
the right and bring your left arm up and over the
top of his, and strike down with your hand into
the elbow hinge, pulling him down and forward
and throwing him off balance. Your response
must be lightning-quick, because the movement
of drawing him forward also means that his
punching arm is coming closer to you.

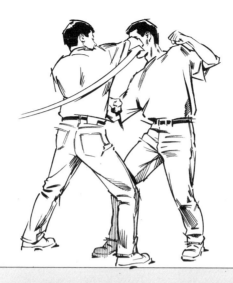

Keep your face down and out of the way during the movement. His head will have been brought down and into a perfect position for your right elbow to come up to his face.

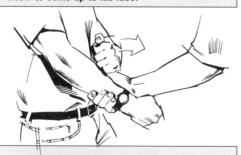

A simple but effective way of defeating a grab is to bend back an attacker's finger or thumb, which will inflict a lot of pain.

Self-defence techniques

Defeating a front grab with a head lock

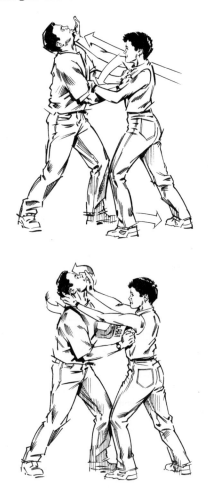

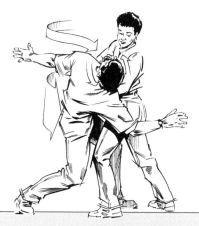

Where the head goes, so does the rest of the body. So if you can control an attacker's head, you can use it to put him down on the ground, without using a great deal of strength. Before you can turn the head, though, you need to push it right back, otherwise the neck muscles will be too strong for you to overcome. So in this case, when an attacker grabs you from the front, swing your left arm up and over the top, bringing it down on the hinge of his right arm. Come in with your right palm and drive it into his chin, pushing the head right back (opposite, top left). Step forward and grab the back of his head with your left arm, as you keep pushing back with your right (opposite, bottom left). Now shove his chin to your left, pulling the back of his head towards you and down at the same time. Control his head around and down, to your left, forcing him on to the ground and onto his back (above).

Self-defence techniques

Defeating a front grab with a wrist lock

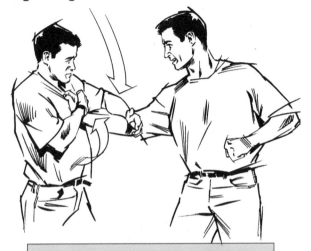

There are various locks that you can apply to the wrist, but this one makes use of your opponent's thumb as a lever as well. However, a word of caution. Applying a lock successfully takes many hours of hard practice, sometimes hundreds of hours. Do not attempt a lock of any kind unless you are absolutely sure that it is necessary and that it will work. Remember, while you are busy applying a lock the attacker has another free arm, and while locks can be extremely painful and disabling, if not applied quickly you could find yourself being struck by the other hand. Decide whether you really need to apply a lock. If your assailant needs restraining for any reason, then a lock is called for. But if your aim is to flee, it is unnecessary.

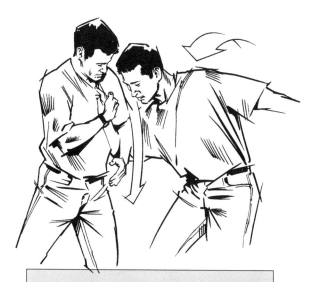

Assume your attacker has grabbed you with his right hand. Bring your own left arm up over his, and pull down into his elbow and towards you. This will help break his grip and unbalance him as he is pulled towards you. Bring your right hand up and grab his fingers. Push his hand back against his wrist, and bring your left hand up to trap his thumb. Remember that all this must be performed in a split-second to be successful. When used in a self-defence scenario all these moves will be combined into one fluid movement. You must have practised long and hard for this move. You must give your attacker no time in which to recover before you apply the lock – if you make a mistake you will not get a second chance.

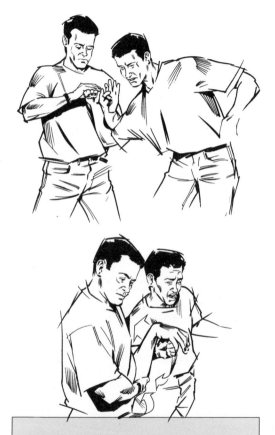

Bring your right hand up and grab his fingers, and bring your left hand up and trap his thumb (top). Drop your right hand down to his elbow and pull it down and towards you (above).

Defence against bear hug 1

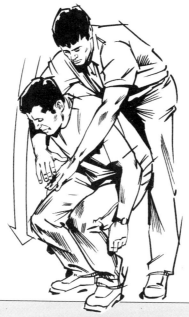

If you get grabbed from behind in a bear hug, do not try to struggle free in an upright position. The chances are that you will not be able to break away and you will just tire yourself out. Rather, while your arms are trapped, drop your weight down and forward as far as you can. If you do this quickly enough, you can drop out of an attacker's grip. This is particularly effective if you are a stocky person, as all of a sudden your attacker has to try to hold up your entire body weight rather than let it drop.

Self-defence techniques

Defence against bear hug 2

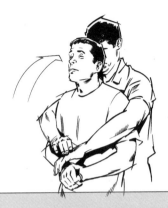

If an attacker is holding you too tightly, then snap your head back as hard as you can, butting him in the face. At the same time, try to rip away at any of his fingers to inflict pain.

Defence against bear hug 3

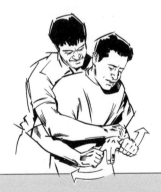

If your arms are free, you can still execute a head butt, but it may be easier for you to grab your attacker's fingers and rip them apart.

Defence against bear hug 4

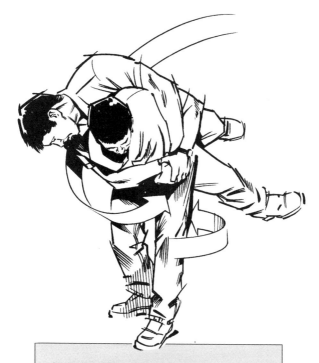

As an alternative, if you are confident about your own strength, and your attacker is not significantly heavier than you, you can drop your weight down a little, bend forward to bring him up and forward, grip his arms tightly, then straighten your legs and twist at the same time. If you have unbalanced him, you will throw him over your hip and onto the floor.

Defence against strangles

Defence techniques against strangles are similar to those used to defeat grabs, combining speed and blows to free yourself.

Defence against a two-handed strangle

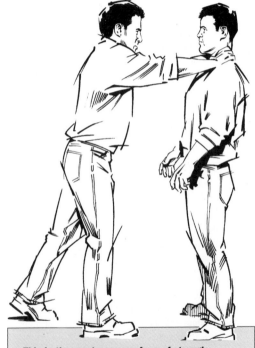

This is the most common form of strangle attack, especially in attacks against women and in domestic violence situations. For that reason, you must know how to defeat it.

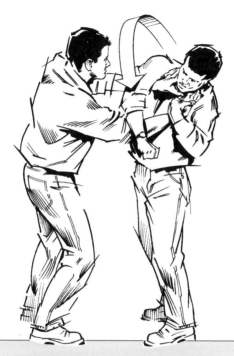

It is very important to counterattack against a strangle as quickly as possible. Remember that strangling cuts off the supply of blood and/or oxygen to the brain. It is therefore potentially fatal. You may only have seconds in which to react before you slip into unconsciousness, and then death. Therefore, relax your neck as much possible (it makes it harder for an attacker to get an effective strangle). Throw your weight violently to one side (in this case the left), bringing your right arm up and over his.

Self-defence techniques

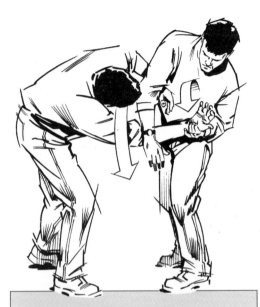

After you have thrown your weight to one side, reach up and take his right hand with your left. As you keep turning, the pressure of your right arm is putting a lock on his left, which will cause him to let go. (Note: If you are very small in stature and are being strangled by a large, powerful attacker, it may be impractical to throw your weight to one side. In this case you will have to improvise. Try collapsing to the ground; however strong your adversary, will he be able to hold up your entire body weight with his arms outstretched? An attacker with his arms around your neck is not protecting his groin. If this area is within reach, try a kick – he will release his grip if you make contact!)

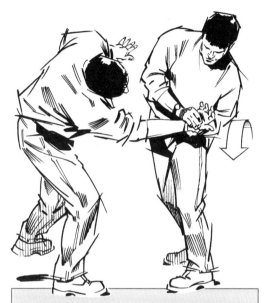

Following on from the move opposite, turn your
attacker's right wrist out, putting a lock on
it. With both his arms trapped, he is now in a
perfect position for you to drive your right elbow
back into his face. Alternatively, you may be in
a position to deliver a downward elbow strike.
Lift your right arm up high with the palm of your
hand facing away from you. Pull your elbow
down rapidly, aiming the point of the elbow at
the spine, rib cage or neck. Do not forget to
throw your weight into the blow, from which
your attacker is unlikely to recover.

Self-defence techniques

Defence against a rear choke

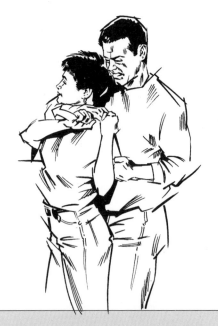

The first rule of self-defence is not to let anyone get close behind you in a threatening situation. But if someone has managed this, and is attacking you with a choke, the first thing to do is relax your neck. This actually makes it harder for the strangle to go on, while the surprise can cause the attacker to momentarily relax his grip (he may think you are unconscious or even dead). Reach up and grab a finger – the little one is usually easiest – and yank it away from you violently to loosen his grip further.

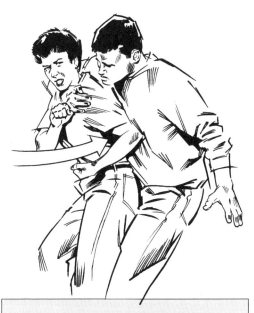

Continue to bend the finger back as far as you can – the pain will cause him to release his grip even more. Then drive back with your elbow into his stomach. You can combine this with stamping down to the rear: you should either get a foot or a shin. If you are wearing stiletto heels, this can be doubly painful to the attacker. In addition, you could attempt a rear head butt: bring your head forward slightly and then snap it back into the attacker's face. A combination attack against an attacker's face, stomach and legs will be more than enough to release the strangle. In addition, your assailant will hopefully not be physically able to resume his assault on you.

Self-defence techniques

Defence against a head lock

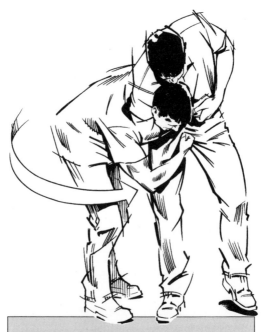

If an attacker has managed to grip your head
and neck under his arm, you need to get out
quickly. If you are facing him, punch your arm
up hard into his groin. If you are alongside him,
facing the same way, you can bring your arm
up between his legs from behind and strike his
genitals. At the same time, bring your other
hand up over the front or top of your head, and
push your own head back as you pull back with
your own body weight; this will release his grip.

Defence on the ground against a two-handed strangle

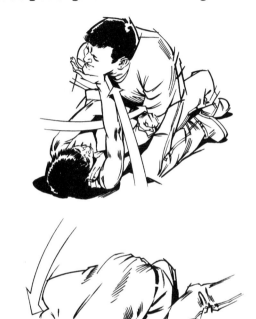

Bring one arm up and over his, and smash down on his elbow hinge, releasing the pressure, then strike into his face with your palm. If you bring his head down close enough, grab his hair, pull him down, and bite into his ear.

Defence against a baton

The first rule concerning defence against weapons is to avoid them at all costs, though it is prudent to be able to deal with them.

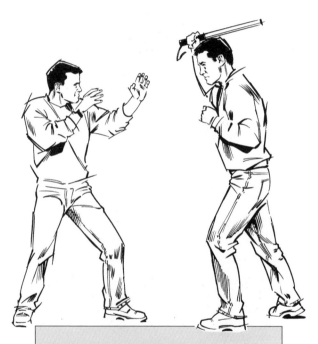

If someone is attacking you with a baton or club, they will most likely try to swing it down onto your head. You need to move in towards the attack, as moving back just allows the attacker time to build up power behind the attack, preventing you from countering.

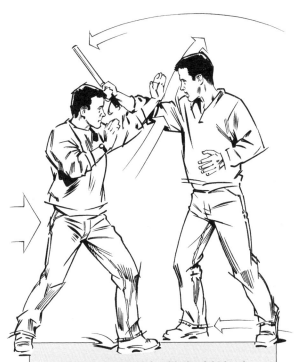

In this case the attack is with the right hand. As he swings, step in and to the right, so that the strike comes down to your left and misses. Block with your left arm as well, although this should not be the main defence. (Note: do not become transfixed by the weapon like a rabbit dazzled by a car's headlights. You must retain your sense of purpose, which is to defeat the attack and disable the attacker. That is why it is important to practise, to familiarise yourself with what the move entails.)

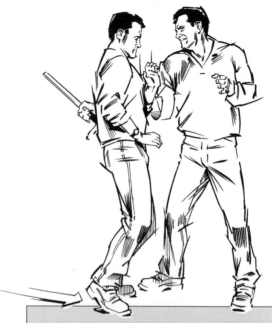

Your left arm should now shoot up and past
his head. Continue the movement around his
arm, bringing your forearm and hand under his
arm and up across your body. You should have
trapped his arm against your body, while taking
his balance at the same time. If you are lucky
you'll be putting pressure on his elbow, too. The
weapon is now harmless and you are free to
launch a counter strike. Having trapped his arm,
not only will have rendered the weapon safe,
you will also be inflicting considerable pain on
your attacker, giving you the initiative to further
disable him.

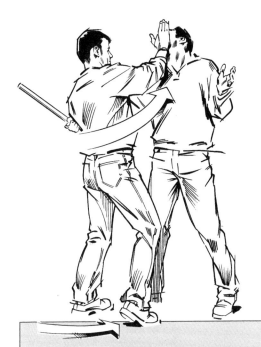

This is the final part of the movement. His head will be slightly forward, and wide open for a strike. So step and twist forward, driving up into his chin with the heel of your right palm (or an upper cut with your right elbow if you prefer). if you strike slightly across to the left, this will take his balance further, and he will fall back and to the left. Note the position of your legs in relation to his groin. The attacker is wide open to a groin strike with your right knee. This will undoubtedly finish him off and put him on the ground.

Defence against knives

The following techniques for dealing with knives should only be used as a last resort. Knife attacks tend to be erratic and frenzied. Beware!

Defence against overhead stab

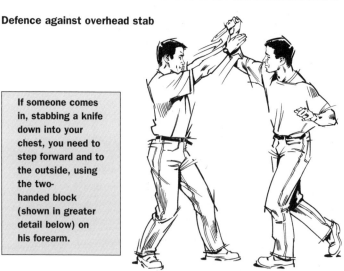

If someone comes in, stabbing a knife down into your chest, you need to step forward and to the outside, using the two-handed block (shown in greater detail below) on his forearm.

The cross block

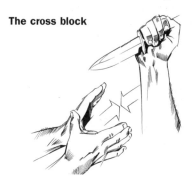

With the cross block, you don't cross your forearms, but rather have both thumbs open and overlapping the other hand. Try to catch the arm as close to the hand as possible.

Once you've blocked the knife thrust, keep hold of the forearm, twist your body sharply to the right and bring the attacker's arm down quickly, throwing him off-balance as you do.

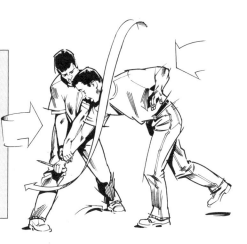

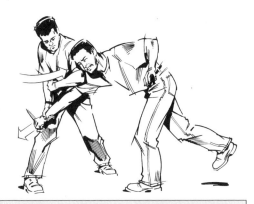

From here, you can drive your left elbow up and into his face. Alternatively, when you come in with the cross block, stop his arm while it is still in the air and knee him in the groin.

Self-defence techniques

Defence against underhand stab 1

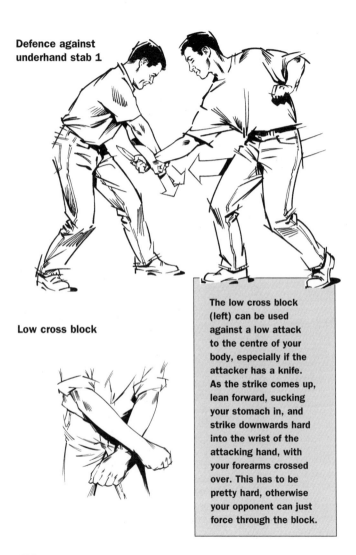

Low cross block

The low cross block (left) can be used against a low attack to the centre of your body, especially if the attacker has a knife. As the strike comes up, lean forward, sucking your stomach in, and strike downwards hard into the wrist of the attacking hand, with your forearms crossed over. This has to be pretty hard, otherwise your opponent can just force through the block.

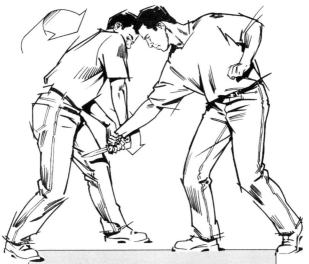

I am right handed, so I have my right arm over my left, but you can do it the other way around. If you keep your hands open, you can grab his hand before turning into a wrist or arm lock. If an underhand knife strike is coming in to your stomach, you need to use the low cross block shown on the opposite page. Pull your stomach in, lean forward and drive your hands down into the attacker's wrist. You should have the forearms crossed, with your right over your left. Remember to make the block forceful, so that your assailant can't just push past it. Slide your hand around the back of his hand then twist it up and around. Now your other hand should also take a grip, again with the thumb in the back of his hand. By this time his fingers should be pointing upwards.

Self-defence techniques

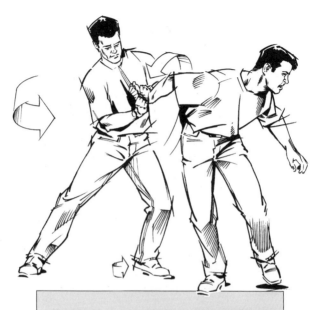

You should now press back, forcing his wrist into a right angle with his arm, or further if it will go. Keep turning the hand around, forcing his elbow up and applying a painful lock.

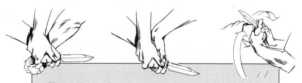

These three diagrams show the positioning of the hands, fingers and thumbs when twisting an attacker's knife hand while carrying out the techniques illustrated on pages 139 to 141.

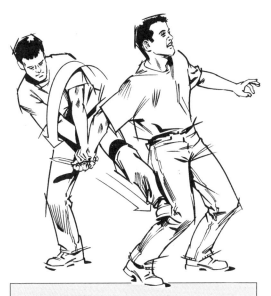

Once you have your attacker's knife hand back as far as it will go, you can launch a stamping kick into the back or side of his knee, forcing him down to the ground. Alternatively, once you have the wrist twisted around, you can pull back and down, all the time keeping the pressure on the wrist. This will unbalance him and force him to the ground. Once he is on the ground, you may consider keeping hold of his wrist and twisting it to dislocate the arm. This may sound brutal, but remember that the attacker had the intention of seriously hurting you, even killing you. You cannot afford the risk of him getting off the ground and launching another attack against you.

Self-defence techniques

Defence against underhand stab 2

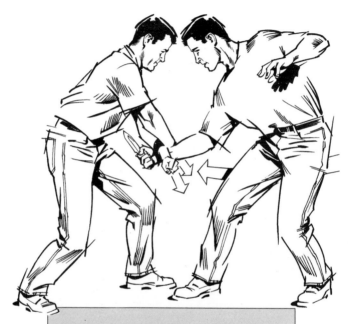

This is a variation on the defence technique
shown on pages 138 to 141. Once you have
the wrist twisted round, you can pull back and
down, all the time keeping the pressure on the
wrist. This will unbalance the attacker and force
him to the ground. But I must emphasise that
the first rule of fighting someone with a knife is
don't do it. The damage a knife can do, even in
the hands of an unskilled novice, is immense. It
can kill you.

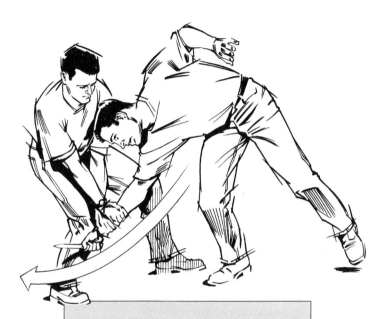

If someone wants your wallet or handbag, and he is waving a knife at you, my advice would be to hand over the money. But if you can't escape, and someone is determined to stab or slash you, then the techniques shown above can help. But be warned. Reading a book like this is not enough. And you must expect to get cut – even the most skilled martial artist doesn't face down a knife unless he has no other choice.

Self-defence in cars

Being able to deal with unwelcome intruders in your vehicle is very important, especially for lone women drivers and the elderly.

Knife hand to the neck

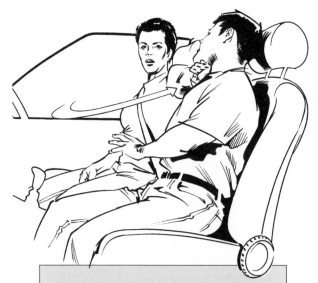

> If you are a lone driver who is attacked in a car, especially if you are a woman, you need to attract attention and get help quickly. Flash the lights, hit the hazard flashers or the horn, drive into another car, do anything rather than let him get you away to a secluded spot.
> If the car is stopped, and the attacker is sitting alongside you, you can chop up into his throat using the side of your hand.

Elbow strike

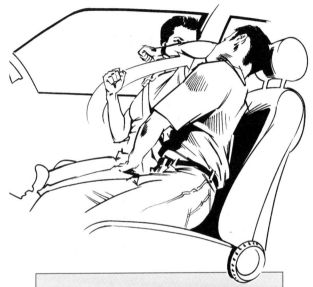

If an attacker is closer, then use your elbow against his face rather than your hand. You need to wind your body up and twist from the hips to get your full weight and force behind the strike (it doesn't matter how small you are). Drive your elbow into his chin or face. You can also strike into the jaw. Remember that you will have your seat belt on and your attacker will have more freedom of movement than you. Therefore, as soon as someone who is not welcome enters your vehicle, strike immediately to defend yourself (as a matter of course you should drive with all your doors locked).

Self-defence techniques

Defence against a rear strangle in a vehicle

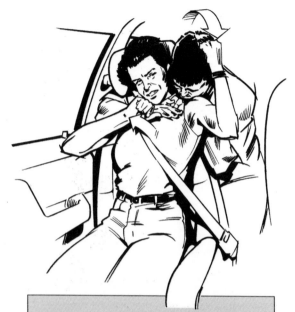

If the attacker is in the seat behind you, he will normally either try to throw his arms around you, or choke you with his hands. Either way you have got to act fast. So, as with any standard grabbing attack, go for any finger you can reach and bend it back as hard as you can. This will cause your assailant extreme pain. If you can reach, bend your other arm back and try to find his hair. Pulling it forward will cause him pain. If you can't grab his hair for any reason, try jabbing behind with your fingers in an effort to attack his eyes.

Removing an unwelcome visitor from your car

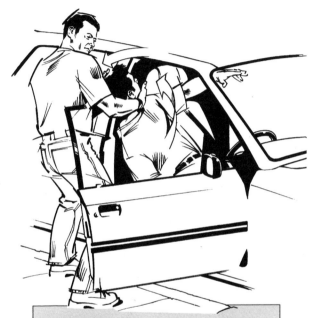

You may be in a situation when someone hostile is sitting in your car and you want to get him out. This can be difficult, because of his weight, and if he is in the driving seat he can hang on to the wheel or console. So make sure the seat belt is released, then reach in, put two fingers up the nostrils and pull the head back, then lift up. The pain will make him bring his head up, and where his head comes so does the rest of him. You should be able to control him up and out of the car.

Sexual harassment

Being able to fight off sexually motivated attacks and sexual harassment is essential for women and men in today's society.

Unwelcome arms around the shoulder

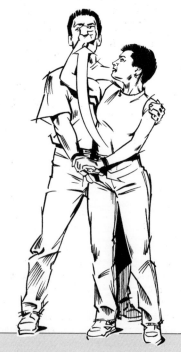

The man is standing alongside with his arm round your shoulder. Snap your own arm up, and smash the back of your fist into his nose. If he continues, turn and head butt him in the face.

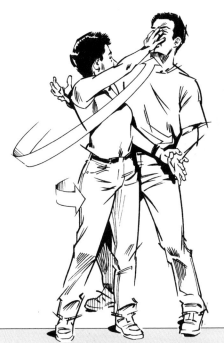

This is an alternative strike when a woman receives unwelcome attention in a bar or club, or even in the street, and a man is standing alongside and putting his arm round her shoulder. If the man is standing to your left and has his right arm round your shoulder, swing round quickly with the other arm and jab your fingers into his eyes. Remember to use the motion of the hips to increase the force of the blow. The finger jab should be enough, but if it isn't you are in an ideal position to deliver a knee strike to his groin.

Self-defence techniques

Countering a bag snatch

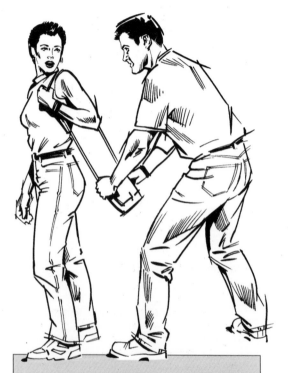

If you carry a shoulder bag, it can be a tempting target for a thief or mugger. Here the situation is someone trying to grab a bag off your shoulder from behind. Though he has crept up on you unawares, the grab has alerted you to his presence. He is now very vulnerable to a number of self-defence strikes.

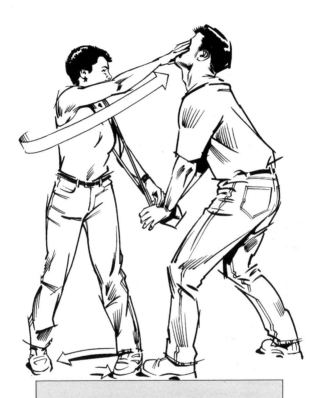

Pivot in towards the thief and strike with the other hand, ideally with a finger jab to the eyes. The shock should make him let go and give you a chance to escape. Alternatively, if he is closer, you can use a palm strike or even a head butt to the face. Remember, if you are carrying a heavy bag, it is a weapon in its own right.

Self-defence techniques

Defence against rape attack

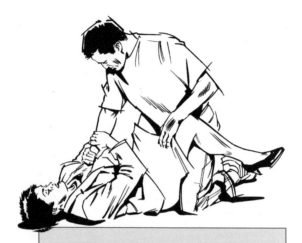

An attacker is on top of you trying to rape you, and has his right hand across your throat (above). Put both your hands on the attacker's wrist and arm to try to ease the pressure on your throat.

Raise your left leg over the attacker's head and bring it in front of his throat. Keep the knee slightly bent, and then force him to your left side with your left leg (opposite top).

As you continue to push him with your left leg, pull his right arm towards you and move your hips towards him so that his elbow is across your hips. As you continue to push with your leg, lift your hips off the ground and pull down his right arm sharply. Keep his right hand close to your throat – this will result in a very painful arm lock (opposite bottom).

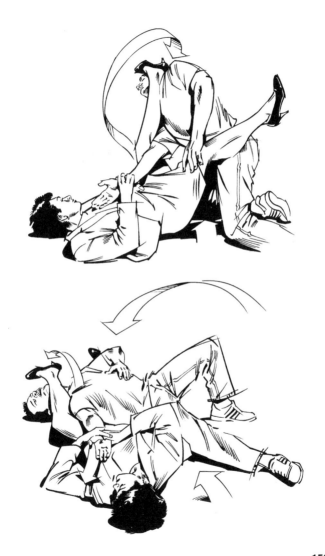

The SAS five-second knockout

The following five illustrations represent a tried and tested method of defeating an attacker in a five-second sequence, as used by the SAS.

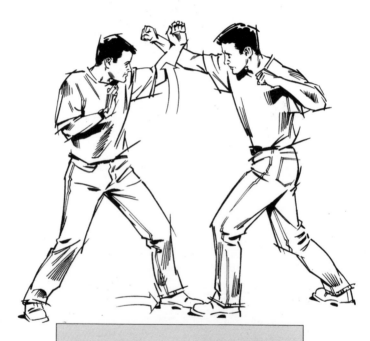

Single techniques are not enough: you need to combine them in to a rapid series of moves, keeping your attacker off balance and winning the fight as quickly as you can. If attacked with a right-handed punch, block with your left arm.

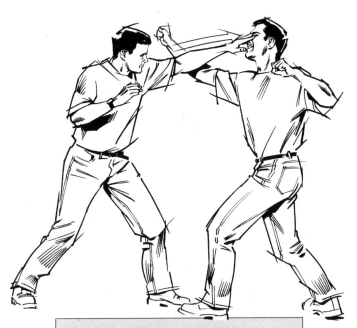

Keep the left arm moving, step inside and forward and go straight in with a left finger jab to the eyes. Resist the temptation to stop the move at this point. The SAS five-second knockout is a quick, reliable and effective way of doing so. You must practise it until it becomes instinctive, then you will view it as one move, rather than a series. Don't forget your training: take up the relaxed, balanced stance described above, and keep aware of what's going on around you at all times.

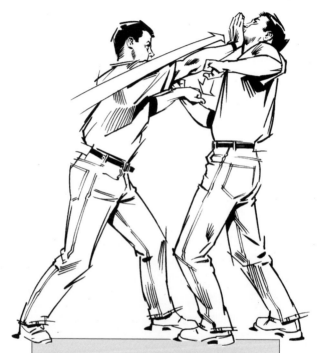

The finger jab to the eyes should have stopped your opponent in his tracks. At the very least it will distract him and leave him wide open for the rest of the sequence. But you must train to perform the whole sequence as a matter of course. Follow up with a right palm heel to the face, which should take his balance and may put him on the ground.

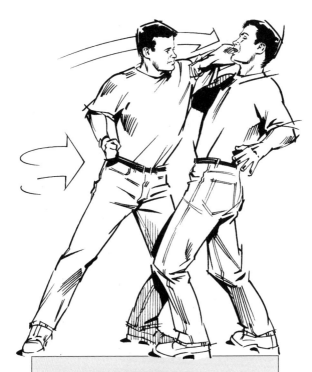

If the attacker hasn't collapsed in a heap on the floor, then step in with your left leg and swing up with your left elbow. The strike should ideally be to the chin, but the side of the face will do. Remember to swing the hips to add to the momentum of the strike: effective weight transferral is much more effective than brute strength in self-defence.

Self-defence techniques

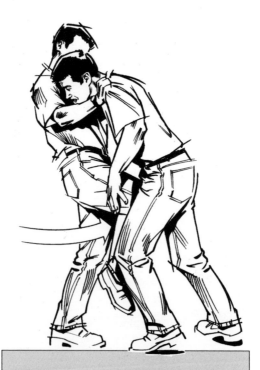

If the attacker hasn't gone down by now, slide
your foot forward and bring your other knee up
into his groin. This will undoubtedly remove any
hostile intentions he may have had towards you.
So, remember the SAS five-second knockout:
block, eyes, palm, elbow, knee. It's been tried
and it works. But remember also that the best
self-defence technique is avoiding trouble.

INDEX

Index